Student Study Guide to Accompany DRUGS AND SOCIETY

Twelfth Edition

Glen R. Hanson
Professor, Department of Pharmacology and Toxicology
Associate Dean, School of Dentistry
Director, Utah Addiction Center
University of Utah
Salt Lake City, Utah
Senior Advisor, National Institute on Drug Abuse
National Institutes of Health
Bethesda, Maryland

Peter J. Venturelli
Chair and Associate Professor,
Department of Sociology and Criminology
Valparaiso University
Valparaiso, Indiana

Annette E. Fleckenstein
Professor, Department of Pharmacology and Toxicology
University of Utah
Salt Lake City, Utah

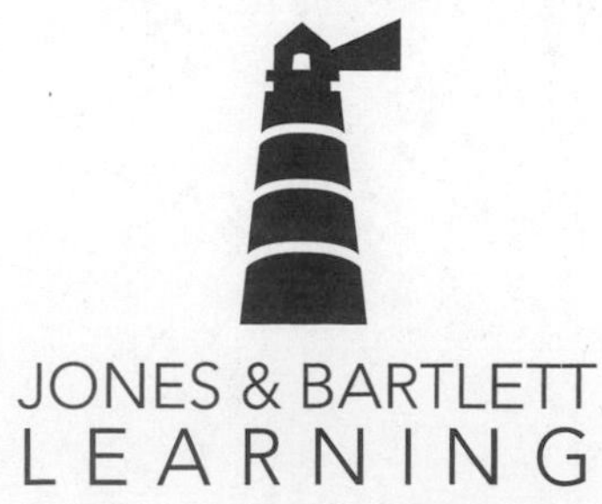

JONES & BARTLETT
LEARNING

World Headquarters
Jones & Bartlett Learning
5 Wall Street
Burlington, MA 01803
978-443-5000
info@jblearning.com
www.jblearning.com

Jones & Bartlett Learning books and products are available through most bookstores and online booksellers. To contact Jones & Bartlett Learning directly, call 800-832-0034, fax 978-443-8000, or visit our website, www.jblearning.com.

Substantial discounts on bulk quantities of Jones & Bartlett Learning publications are available to corporations, professional associations, and other qualified organizations. For details and specific discount information, contact the special sales department at Jones & Bartlett Learning via the above contact information or send an email to specialsales@jblearning.com.

Production Credits
Executive Publisher: William Brottmiller
Publisher: Cathy L. Esperti
Editorial Assistant: Jillian Porazzo
Associate Director of Production: Julie C. Bolduc
Production Editor: Jill Morton
Production Assistant: Brooke Appe
Senior Marketing Manager: Andrea DeFronzo
VP, Manufacturing and Inventory Control: Therese Connell
Composition: Cenveo Publisher Services
Cover Design: Kristin E. Parker
Photo Research and Permissions Coordinator: Amy Rathburn
Cover and Title Page Image: Background, © Eky Studio/ShutterStock, Inc.;
A rocks glass, © Yeko Photo Studio/ShutterStock, Inc.;
Three pills, © Maksud/ShutterStock, Inc.;
An iced coffee, © Yeko Photo Studio/ShutterStock, Inc.;
Rolling a joint, © Nikita Starichenko/ShutterStock, Inc.;
Steroids used by an athlete, © Jupiterimages/liquidlibrary/Thinkstock;
An aisle of pills, © Jupiterimages/Photos.com/Thinkstock;
A spray can, © Mikael Damkier/ShutterStock, Inc.;
A cigarette, © Mariusz Szachowski/ShutterStock, Inc.;
A drug user, © iStockphoto/Thinkstock
Printing and Binding: Edwards Brother Malloy
Cover Printing: Edwards Brother Malloy

ISBN: 978-1-284-03548-3

6048
Printed in the United States of America
18 17 16 15 14 10 9 8 7 6 5 4 3 2

Contents

Introduction

The impact of drug use and/or abuse on the lives of ordinary people is a topic that is important and complex enough to study for an entire semester. For some students this course is necessary to fulfill degree requirements for graduation; others choose it as an elective. Most students are surprised at the volume of information covered in a course on drugs and society and sometimes do not appreciate the multiple dimensions and body of knowledge until after the first quiz or exam.

Each of us brings unique backgrounds, experiences, values, and beliefs to discussions of drug issues. These factors influence our decision-making in a variety of ways. In this course, you will gain a real perspective of drug-related problems in our society. No matter your discipline, in this course, you will find useful current information and perspectives to help you understand:

- Social and psychological reasons why drug use and abuse occur
- The results of drug use and abuse on body/brain functions and behavior
- How to prevent drug use and abuse
- How drugs can be used effectively for therapeutic purposes
- Current major drug abuse patterns and their causes

The knowledge gained in this course can both protect and enhance your life and the lives of those with whom you associate.

This study guide is designed to help you organize and reinforce your learning about the issues covered in *Drugs and Society, Twelfth Edition.* The following features can be found in each of the chapters:

- **Chapter Outlines** Provide an organizational guide to the topics and ideas presented in each chapter.
- **Self-Tests** Test your knowledge of the reading and give you a chance to revisit concepts. Each chapter contains all or some of the following: Key Terms, Fill-in-the-Blank, Identify, Matching, True/False, and Discussion Questions.
- **Lecture Slides** Help you to have organized notes, which is essential when completing assignments and at exam time.

Lecture Slides

The lecture slide component is located at the end of each chapter and contains the full set of the PowerPoint presentations that accompany your textbook as well as space next to each slide for you to jot down the terms and concepts you feel are most important to each lecture. This guide will save you from having to write down everything on the slides. Do the assigned reading, listen in lecture, follow the key points your instructor makes, and write down meaningful notes. This is the perfect place to write down questions you want to ask your professor later or reminders to study a concept again to make sure you really got it. For more information on the most effective note-taking methods that will save you both time and effort when reviewing for exams, see the Note-Taking Tips.

Once the lecture slide component of this Study Guide has helped to organize and simplify your notes on each chapter, the self-tests will assess how well you have mastered the material. Your ability to easily locate the important concepts of a recent lecture and test yourself on the most important points and terminology will prove to be essential at exam time.

This Study Guide is a valuable resource. You've found a wonderful study partner!

Note-Taking Tips

1. It is easier to take notes if you are not hearing the information for the first time. Read the chapter or the material that is about to be discussed before class. This will help you to anticipate what will be said in class, and have an idea of what to write down. It will also help to read over your notes from the last class. This way you can avoid having to spend the first few minutes of class trying to remember where you left off last time.
2. Don't waste your time trying to write down everything that your professor says. Instead, listen closely and only write down the important points. Review these important points after class to help remind you of related points that were made during the lecture.
3. If the class discussion takes a spontaneous turn, pay attention and participate in the discussion. Only take notes on the conclusions that are relevant to the lecture.
4. Emphasize main points in your notes. You may want to use a highlighter, special notation (asterisks, exclamation points), format (circle, underline), or placement on the page (indented, bulleted). You will find that when you try to recall these points, you will be able to actually picture them on the page.
5. Be sure to copy down word-for-word specific formulas, laws, and theories.
6. Hearing something repeated, stressed, or summed up can be a signal that it is an important concept to understand.
7. Organize handouts, study guides, and exams in your notebook along with your lecture notes. It may be helpful to use a three-ring binder, so that you can insert pages wherever you need to.
8. When taking notes, you might find it helpful to leave a wide margin on all four sides of the page. Doing this allows you to note names, dates, definitions, etc., for easy access and studying later. It may also be helpful to make notes of questions you want to ask your professor about or research later, ideas or relationships that you want to explore more on your own, or concepts that you don't fully understand.
9. It is best to maintain a separate notebook for each class. Labeling and dating your notes can be helpful when you need to look up information from previous lectures.
10. Make your notes legible, and take notes directly in your notebook. Chances are you won't recopy them no matter how noble your intentions. Spend the time you would have spent recopying the notes studying them instead, drawing conclusions and making connections that you didn't have time for in class.
11. Look over your notes after class while the lecture is still fresh in your mind. Fix illegible items and clarify anything you don't understand. Do this again right before the next class.

CHAPTER 1

Introduction to Drugs and Society

Chapter Outline

The chapter outline provides you with an organizational guide to the topics and ideas presented in this chapter of the text.

Key Terms

Define the following terms:

1. **Insiders/Outsiders** ____________________
2. **Drugs** ____________________
3. **Opioids** ____________________
4. **Addiction** ____________________
5. **Gateway drugs** ____________________

6. **Licit/illicit/OTC drugs** ______________________________

7. **Designer drugs/synthetic drugs or synthetic opioids** ______________________________

8. **Equal-opportunity affliction** ______________________________

9. **Employee Assistance Programs (EAPs)** ______________________________

■ Fill-in-the-Blank

1. ______________________________ are drugs that result from altered chemical structures of current illicit drugs.

2. The unintentional or inappropriate use of prescribed or over-the-counter (OTC) types of drugs is known as ______________________________.

3. ______________________________ refers to the need to continue taking a drug to avoid withdrawal symptoms.

4. ______________________________ are drug compounds that affect the central nervous system and alter consciousness and/or perceptions.

5. Coffee, tea, alcohol, tobacco, and over-the-counter drugs are all examples of ______________ drugs. Marijuana, cocaine, and LSD are all ______________ drugs.

6. ______________________________ are new drugs that are developed by people intending to circumvent the illegality of a drug by modifying a drug into a new compound. An example of this kind of drug is ______________________.

7. The ______________________ is the principal federal agency for enforcing U.S. drug laws.

8. Drug testing may be administered in three ways:

a. ______________________________

b. ______________________________

c. ______________________________

■ Identify

1. Identify the three categories of drug users and explain the characteristics of each.

a. ______________________________

b. ______________________________

c. ______________________________

2. Identify and describe the five phases of addiction.

a. ______________________________

b. ______________________________

c. ______________________________

d. ______________________________

e. ______________________________

3. Identify the four principal factors that affect drug use and explain each one.

a. ______________________________

b. ______________________________

c. ______________________________

d. ______________________________

4. Identify the four main characteristics necessary for drug dependence.

a. ______________________________

b. ______________________________

c. ______________________________

d. ______________________________

5. Identify and define Erich Goode's four types of drug use.

a. ______________________________

b. ______________________________

c. ______________________________

d. ______________________________

6. Identify five reasons why people take drugs.

a. ______________________________

b. ______________________________

c. ______________________________

d. ______________________________

e. ______________________________

Discussion Questions

1. Give three examples of drug misuse.

2. Why do Americans use so many legal drugs (for example, alcohol, tobacco, and OTC drugs)? What aspects of our society promote extensive drug use?

3. What do you believe is the relationship between excessive drug use and crime? Does drug use *cause* crime or is crime simply a manifestation of personality?

4. Describe the holistic self-awareness approach to drug use. Discuss your thoughts on this approach and its effectiveness in drug abuse treatment.

5. How do you think drug use is different today in comparison to ancient historical times?

Notes

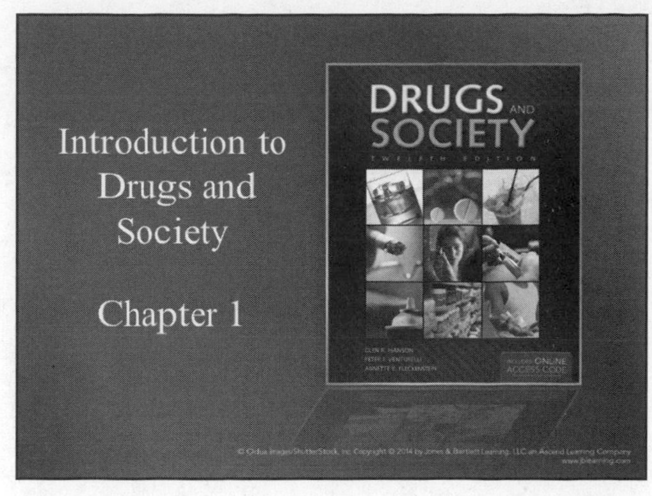

Key Concerns

- What constitutes a drug?
- What are the most commonly abused drugs?
- What are designer drugs?
- How widespread is drug use?
- What is the extent and frequency of drug use in our society?
- What are the current statistics and trends in drug use?

Key Concerns (continued)

- What types of drug users exist?
- How does the media influence drug use?
- What attracts people to drug use?
- When does drug use lead to drug dependence?
- When does drug addiction occur?
- What are the costs of drug addiction to society?
- What can be gained by learning about the complexity of drug use and abuse?

Notes

Drug Use Causes Three Major Simultaneous Changes in the User

1. The social and psychological rewards from the effects of the drug "high" results in the illusion of temporary satisfaction and postponement of social pressures and anxieties leading to a superficial belief that problems and/or concerns are nonproblematic.
2. Pharmacologically, the nonmedical use of most drugs alters body chemistry largely by interfering with (affecting) its proper (homeostatic) functioning. Drugs enhance, slow down, speed-up, or distort the reception and transmission of reality.
3. Using a particular drug may satisfy an inborn or genetically programmed need or desire.

Drug Use

- Drug users are found in all occupations and professions, at all income and social class levels, and in all age groups.
- No one is immune to drug use, (that often leads to drug dependence). Drug use is an *equal-opportunity affliction.*

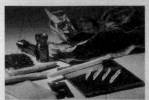

Examples of illicit drugs that can become costly once drug dependence occurs.

© Comstock Images/Getty Images

Four Principle Factors That Affect Drug Use

- **Biological, Genetic, and Pharmacological Factors:** Substance abuse and addiction involve biological and genetic factors. The pharmacology of drug use focuses on how the ingredients of a particular drug affect the body and the nervous system, and in turn, a person's experience with a particular drug.
- **Cultural Factors:** How do societal views, determined by custom and tradition, affect our initial approach to and use of a drug?
- **Social Factors:** What are the specific reasons why a drug is taken (e.g., curing an illness, self-medicating, escape from reality, peer pressure, family upbringing, membership in drug-abusing subcultures)?
- **Contextual Factors:** How do physical surroundings (music concerts, bars, nightclubs, or fraternity and sorority parties) affect the amount of drug use?

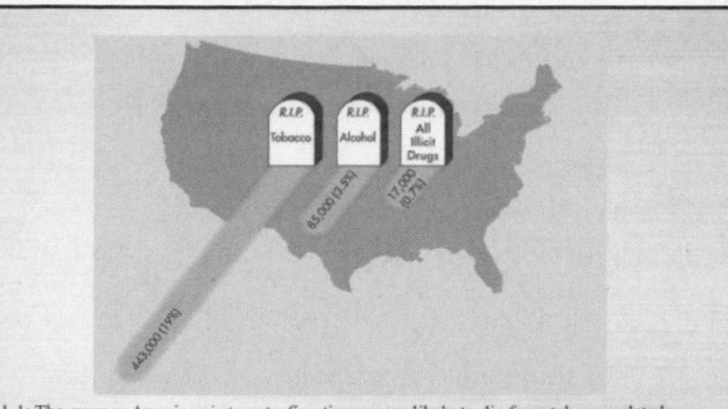

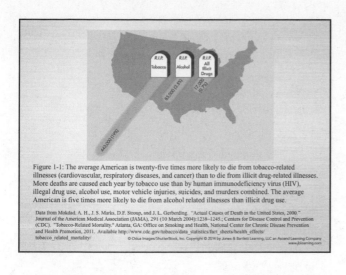

Figure 1-1: The average American is twenty-five times more likely to die from tobacco-related illnesses (cardiovascular, respiratory diseases, and cancer) than to die from illicit drug-related illnesses. More deaths are caused each year by tobacco use than by human immunodeficiency virus (HIV), illegal drug use, alcohol use, motor vehicle injuries, suicides, and murders combined. The average American is five times more likely to die from alcohol related illnesses than illicit drug use.

Data from Mokdad, A. H., J. S. Marks, D.F. Stroup, and J. L. Gerberding. "Actual Causes of Death in the United States, 2000." Journal of the American Medical Association (JAMA), 291 (10 March 2004):1238–1245.; Centers for Disease Control and Prevention (CDC). "Tobacco-Related Mortality." Atlanta, GA: Office on Smoking and Health, National Center for Chronic Disease Prevention and Health Promotion, 2011. Available http://www.cdc.gov/tobacco/data_statistics/fact_sheets/health_effects/tobacco_related_mortality/

The Dimensions of Drug Abuse

Q: What is a drug?
A: Any substance that modifies (enhances, inhibits, or distorts) mind and/or body functioning.

Q: What are psychoactive drugs?
A: Drug compounds (substances) that affect the central nervous system and/or alter consciousness and/or perceptions.

Psychoactive Drugs

- Psychoactive drugs are classified as either:
  - **Licit (Legal):** Examples may include coffee, tea, alcohol, tobacco, and over-the-counter drugs.
  - **Illicit (Illegal):** Examples may include marijuana, cocaine, and LSD.

Notes

Notes

Major Types of Commonly Abused Drugs

- Alcohol (ethanol)
- Nicotine (all forms of tobacco)
- Prescription drugs (many drugs that are prescribed by a physician)
- Stimulants
  - Major stimulants: amphetamines, cocaine, and crack
  - Minor stimulants: nicotine, caffeine, tea, and chocolate
- Hallucinogens/psychedelics: LSD, mescaline, peyote, and psilocybin ("magic mushrooms")

Major Types of Commonly Abused Drugs (continued)

- Bath salts (a designer drug)
- Depressants: barbiturates, benzodiazepines, valium, and alcohol
- Cannabis: marijuana and hashish
- Anabolic steroids: a synthetic form of the male hormone testosterone
- Inhalants/organic solvents: inhalants like gasoline, model glue, paint thinner, certain foods, herbs, and vitamins
- Narcotics/opiates: opium, morphine, codeine, and heroin

Designer Drugs/Synthetic Drugs or Synthetic Opioids

- **Structural analogs** are drugs that result from altered chemical structures of current illicit drugs. It involves modifying the basic molecular skeleton of a compound to form a new molecular species.
- **Designer Drugs /Synthetic Drugs or Synthetic Opioids**
  - New categories of hybrid drugs like Ecstasy and Demerol.
  - These relatively recent types of drugs are created as structural analogs of substances already classified under the Controlled Substances Act.

Gateway Drugs

- **Gateway drugs** are types of commonly used drugs that are believed to lead to the use of other more powerful mind-altering and addictive drugs, such as hallucinogens, cocaine, crack, and heroin.
  - Alcohol, tobacco, and marijuana are the most commonly used gateway drugs.

Drug Misuse

- **Drug misuse** is the unintentional or inappropriate use of prescribed or over-the-counter (OTC) types of drugs.

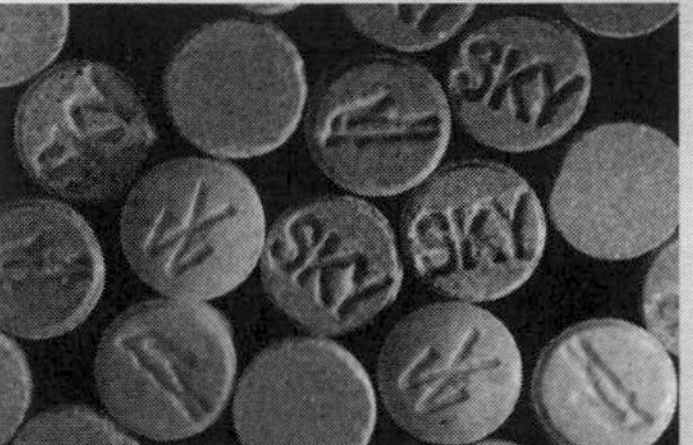

Designer pills made from the illicit drug ecstacy. This drug has some stimulant properties like amphetamines as well as hallucinogens properties like LSD.

Courtesy of DEA.

Six Examples of Drug Misuse

1. Taking more drugs than prescribed
2. Using OTC or psychoactive drugs in excess without medical supervision
3. Mixing drugs with alcohol or other types of drugs
4. Using old medicines to self-treat new symptoms of an illness
5. Discontinuing prescribed drugs at will and/or against physician's orders
6. Administering prescribed drugs to a family member without medical consultation and supervision

Notes

Notes

Dimensions of Drug Abuse

- **Drug abuse** is also known as chemical or substance abuse and is the willful misuse of either licit or illicit drugs for the purpose of recreation, perceived necessity, or convenience.
  - Drug abuse refers to a more intense misuse of drugs—often to the point of addiction.
  - Also known as *chemical* or *substance* abuse.

Erich Goode's Four Types of Drug Use

- **Legal instrumental use:** Taking prescribed drugs or OTC drugs to relieve or treat mental or physical symptoms
- **Legal recreational use:** Using licit drugs like tobacco, alcohol, and caffeine to achieve a certain mental state
- **Illegal instrumental use:** Taking nonprescribed drugs to achieve a task or goal
- **Illegal recreational use:** Taking illicit drugs for fun or pleasure

Drug Use: Statistics and Trends

- **Social Drugs**
  - $90 billion for alcohol
  - $51.9 billion for cigarettes
  - $2 billion for cigars, chewing tobacco, pipe tobacco, roll-your-own tobacco, and snuff
  - $5.7 billion for coffee, teas, and cocoa
- **Prescription Drugs**
  - $950 billion worldwide in 2012.
  - $237.5 billion in the United States

Drug Use: Statistics and Trends (continued)

- **OTC Drugs**
  - $23.5 billion
- **Nonmedical Use of Prescription Drugs**
  - In 2008, 51.9 million Americans age 12 or older had used prescription-type drugs nonmedically at least once in their lifetime.
- **Miscellaneous Drugs**
  - Examples include inhalants, nutmeg, and morning glory seeds
  - Extent of use cannot be verified

Drug Quiz

Q: How many Americans, age 12 and up, have used alcohol in the past month?

A: 125 million

Q: How many Americans in the past month have smoked tobacco?

A: 61.5 million

Drug Quiz (continued)

Q: How many Americans use or have used marijuana/hashish in their lifetime?

A: 107,842 million (41.9%)

Q: How many drugs can be found in the average household?

A: 50 drugs (40% prescriptions, 60% OTC)

Notes

Notes

National Household Survey on Drug Abuse, 2011

- 82.2% (211.7 million) Americans used alcohol during their lifetime
- 62.8 (161.7 million) Americans used cigarettes
- 47% (117 million) Americans used any illicit drug(s)

Most commonly used illicit drugs (Lifetime Use):

- 107.8 million (41.9%) used marijuana/hashish
- 51.3 million (19.9%) used nonmedical use of any psychotherapeutics, such as pain relievers, tranquilizers, stimulants, or sedatives (does not include OTC drugs)
- 36.3 million (14.3%) used cocaine
- 36.3 million (14.4) used hallucinogens
- 34.2 million (13.3%) used pain relievers

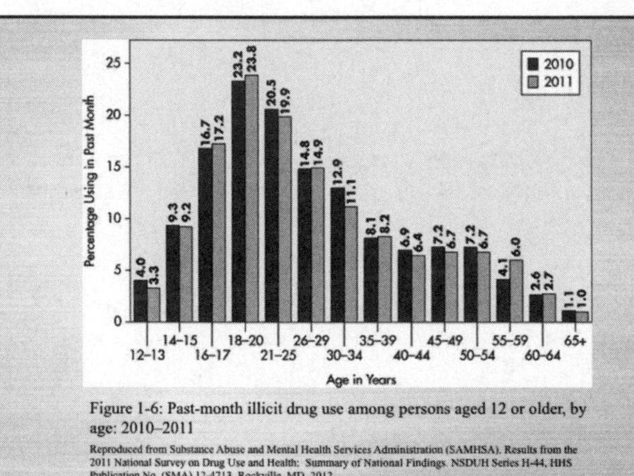

Figure 1-6: Past-month illicit drug use among persons aged 12 or older, by age: 2010–2011

Reproduced from Substance Abuse and Mental Health Services Administration (SAMHSA). Results from the 2011 National Survey on Drug Use and Health: Summary of National Findings. NSDUH Series H-44, HHS Publication No. (SMA) 12-4713. Rockville, MD, 2012.

Drug Use: Additional Findings

Age Patterns: 18–20 age category report the most illicit drug use

Racial and Ethnic Differences: (rates of use, past month, 2002-2011)

Two or more races 13.5%
American Indian/Alaska Natives 13.4%
Black/African American: 10%
Whites: 8.7%
Hispanic or Latino: 8.4%
Asians: 3.8%

Drug Use: Additional Findings (continued)

Gender

- Males were more likely than females among persons age 12 or older to be current illicit drug users (11.1% vs. 6.5%).
- The rate of past-month marijuana use for males was about twice as high for males as the rate for females (9.3% vs. 4.9%).

Pregnant Women

- Pregnant women are less likely to use drugs than similar age women who are not pregnant.

Drug Use: Additional Findings (continued)

Education: College graduates (5.4%) had the lowest rate of current illicit drug use, while those who did not complete high school (11.1%) had the highest use of illicit drugs. Past-month alcohol use increased with higher levels of completed education (35.1% with less than high school vs. 68.2% of college graduates

.**Employment:** Unemployed persons (17.2%) have a greater tendency to use more illicit-types of drugs than people gainfully employed (8% full-time and 11.6% part-time workers).

Drug Use: Additional Findings (continued)

Geography: The rate of past-month illicit drug use was 9.2% in large metropolitan counties, 8.7% in small metropolitan counties, and 5.7% in nonmetropolitan counties.

Criminal Justice: 33% of state prisoners and 25% of federal prisoners reported that they had committed their offenses while under the influence of drugs. In 2008, an estimated 333,000 prisoners were arrested for drug law violations—20% of state and 52% of federal inmates (Sabol and Cooper 2009).

Notes

Notes

Three Types of Drug Users

- **Experimenters:** Begin using drugs largely because of peer pressure and curiosity, and they confine their use to recreational settings
- **Compulsive users:** Devote considerable time and energy into getting high, talk incessantly (sometimes exclusively) about drug use, and become connoisseurs of street drugs
- **Floaters or "chippers":** Focus more on using other people's drugs without maintaining as much of a personal supply

Media Influence on Drug Use

- Each year, the alcohol industry spends more than $1 billion on advertising (television, radio, print, and outdoor ads) (FTC 2007).
- Drug companies spent $1.6 billion a year on televised commercials for Viagra, Claritin, Allegra, and other drugs.
- The advertising budget for Budweiser beer exceeds the entire budget for research on alcoholism and alcohol abusers.
- Alcohol companies spent $4.9 billion on television advertising between 2001 and 2005.
- Teens viewing photos of inebriated friends posted on social media, such as MySpace for example, are four times more likely to have used marijuana and three times more likely to have used alcohol and tobacco.

Why Are People Attracted to Drugs?

People use drugs as a means to temporarily:

- Experience pleasure or heighten good feelings
- Relieve stress, tension, or anxiety
- Forget one's problems and avoid or postpone worries
- Relax after a tension-filled day of work
- Fit in with peers or as a rite of passage
- Enhance religious or mystical experiences
- Relieve pain and some symptoms of illness

When Does Use Lead to Abuse?

- The *amount* of drug taken does not necessarily determine abuse.
- The *motive* for taking the drug is the most important factor in determining presence of abuse.
- Initial drug abuse symptoms include:
  - Excessive use
  - Constant preoccupation about the availability and supply of the drug
  - Refusal to admit excessive use
  - Reliance on the drug

Drug Dependence

Both physical and psychological factors precipitate drug dependence:

- **Physical dependence** refers to the need to continue taking the drug to avoid withdrawal symptoms, which often include feelings of discomfort and illness.
- **Psychological dependence** refers to the need that a user may mentally feel about continuing the use of a drug to experience its effects and/or relieve withdrawal symptoms.

Stages of Drug Dependence

- **Relief:** Satisfaction from negative feelings in using the drug
- **Increased Use:** Involves taking greater quantities of the drug
- **Preoccupation:** Consists of a constant concern with the substance
- **Dependency:** A synonym for addiction, is when more of the drug is sought despite the presence of physical symptoms
- **Withdrawal:** The physical and/or psychological effects from not using the drug

Notes

Notes

Costs of Drug Use to Society

- Illnesses
- Shortened lifespans
- Marital and family strife
- Fetal alcohol syndrome
- Criminalistic behavior
- Drugs in the workplace/disruption of careers and professions
- Cost of assistance programs (e.g., Employee Assistance Programs [EAPs])

Costs of Drug Use to Society: Statistics

- The National Institute on Drug Abuse (NIDA) estimates that the typical narcotic habit costs $100/day.
- A heroin addict must steal three to five times the actual cost of the drugs to maintain a habit—about $100,000 per year.
- Three out of four prostitutes in major cities have a serious drug dependency.

Drugs, Crime, and Violence

Regarding the connection between drug use and crime, the following findings can be summarized:

1. Drug users in comparison to non-drug users are more likely to commit crimes.
2. A high percentage of arrestees are often under the influence of a drug while committing crimes.
3. A high percentage of drug users arrested for drug use and violence are more likely to be under the influence of alcohol and/or stimulant-types of drugs such as cocaine, crack, and methamphetamines.

Drugs in the Workplace

- In the U.S., alcohol and drug use and their related problems costs employers and tax payers billions of dollars per year.
- The National Household surveys found significant drug use in the workplace with 64.3% of full-time workers reported alcohol use (7% to 9% drinking while working) and 6.4% reported marijuana use within the past month (SAMHSA 2012).

Drugs in the Workplace (continued)

- Among the 19 major industry categories, the highest rates of past month illicit drug use among full-time workers aged 18 to 64 were found in accommodations and food services (16.9%), construction (13.7%), and arts, entertainment, and recreation (11.6%); (see Figure 1.10).
- The industry categories with the lowest rates of past month illicit drug use were utilities (3.8%), educational services (4%), and public administration (4.1%).

Drug Testing

- Used to identify those who may be using drugs
- Urine, blood screening, or hair analysis

Duration of Detection /"Cut-Offs" for Urine Analysis:

- Amphetamines: 24–72 hours
- Cocaine/metabolite: 24–72 hours
- Opiates: 24–72 hours
- PCP: 24–96 hours
- THC/metabolite: 24 hours–3 weeks (depends on frequency of use)

Note: Hair analysis 1 to 3 months for all drugs listed above

Notes

Notes

Drug Testing (continued)

- Approximately 70% of large companies, 50% of medium companies, and 22% of small companies drug test.
- Over 90% use urine analysis, less than 20% use blood analysis, and less than 3% use hair analysis.
- Most drug-using youth do not cease drug use when they begin working.

Holistic Self-Awareness Approach

- Holistic philosophy that advocates that the mind, body, and spirit work best when they are drug-free.

CHAPTER 2

Explaining Drug Use and Abuse

■ Chapter Outline

The chapter outline provides you with an organizational guide to the topics and ideas presented in this chapter of the text.

Introduction
Drug Use: A Timeless Affliction
The Origin and Nature of Addiction
- Defining Addiction
- Models of Addiction
- Factors Contributing to Addiction

The Vicious Cycle of Addiction
- Other Nondrug Addictions

Major Theoretical Explanations: Biological
- Abused Drugs as Positive Reinforcers
- Drug Abuse and Psychiatric Disorders
- Genetic Explanations

Major Theoretical Explanations: Psychological
- Distinguishing Between Substance Abuse and Mental Disorders
- The Relationship Between Personality and Drug Use
- Theories Based on Learning Processes
- Social Psychological Learning Theories

Major Theoretical Explanations: Sociological
- Social Influence Theories
- Structural Influence Theories

Danger Signals of Drug Abuse
- Low-Risk and High-Risk Drug Choices

■ Key Terms

Define the following terms:

1. **Self medicating** ______________________________

2. **Moral model** ______________________________

3. **Disease model** ______________________________

4. **Personality disorders** ______________________________

5. **Genetic and biophysicological theories** ______________________________

6. **Social learning theory** ______________________________

7. **Amotivational syndrome** ______________________________

8. **"Double wall" of encapsulation** ______________________________

9. **Neurotransmitters** ______________________________

10. **Habituation** ______________________________

11. **Master status** ______________________________

12. **Subculture theory** ______________________________

13. **Conventional behavior** ______________________________

14. **Control theory** ______________________________

■ Fill-in-the-Blank

1. The belief that people abuse alcohol because they choose to do so defines the ____________ ____________ model of addiction.
2. ____________________ theories explain addiction in terms of genetics, brain dysfunction, and biochemical patterns.
3. The brain transmitter believed to mediate the rewarding aspects of most drugs of abuse is called ____________________.
4. How drug substances alter and affect the brain's mental functions are known as ____________ ____________ effects.
5. People who characteristically are continually seeking new or novel thrills in their experiences are known as ____________________.
6. The ratio between reinforcers, both favorable and unfavorable, for sustaining drug use behavior is called ____________________.
7. ____________________ is the theory emphasizing that other people's perceptions directly influence one's self-image.
8. The process of redefining a person in light of a major status position is known as ____________ ____________.
9. ____________________ is the growth and development process responsible for learning how to become a responsible, functioning human being.

■ Identify

1. The diagnosis of substance use disorder includes the following six factors:

   a. ______________________________

   b. ______________________________

   c. ______________________________

   d. ______________________________

e. ______

f. ______

2. Identify the three major models of addiction and briefly explain the beliefs of each model.

a. ______

b. ______

c. ______

3. Identify five danger signals of drug use.

a. ______

b. ______

c. ______

d. ______

e. ______

■ Discussion Questions

1. Why are drug use and abuse even more serious issues now than they were in the past? Give three possible reasons and discuss their significance. ______

2. Discuss the connection between psychiatric disorders and drug abuse. ______

3. Discuss some risk factors for the development of abuse. ______

4. Explain the major differences between social influence theories and structural influence theories. Give an example of each. ______

5. According to the labeling theory, what are the two phases of deviance? Explain the difference between the two. At what point does a person transition from one type of deviance to the other? What do you think causes this transition? ____

____

____

6. Discuss the importance of making low-risk drug choices. How might one maintain a low-risk approach to drug use? ____

____

____

Notes

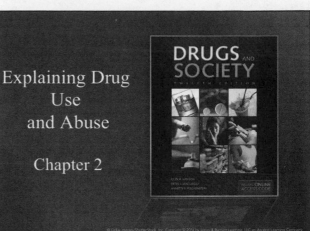

Why Do People Use Drugs?

- What causes people to subject their bodies and minds to the harmful effects of nonmedical and/or recreational drug use that often leads to drug addiction?
- Why is drug use a more serious problem today than in the past?
- Why are some people attracted to recreational drug use?

Ten Reasons Why Drug Use Is More Serious Today

- From 1960 to the present, drug use has become a widespread phenomenon.
- Drugs are much more potent than they were years ago.
- Drug use remains extremely popular. Drugs sales are a multibillion-dollar-a-year business, with major influence on many national economies.
- More so today than years ago, both licit and illicit drugs are experimented with by youths at an increasingly younger age. These drugs are often supplied by older siblings, friends, and acquaintances.

Notes

Ten Reasons Why Drug Use Is More Serious Today (continued)

- Through the media (such as television, radio, magazine, and newspaper advertising), people in today's society are more directly exposed to drug advertising.
- Greater availability and wider dissemination of drug information through emails, drug websites for purchasing prescription drugs without prescriptions, chat rooms, and methods and instructions on how to make drugs.
- Crack as well as crystal methamphetamine and other manufactured "newer" drugs offer potent effects at a low cost.

Ten Reasons Why Drug Use Is More Serious Today (continued)

- Drug use endangers the future of a society by harming its youth and potentially destroying the lives of many young men and women.
- Drug use and especially drug dealing are becoming major factors in the growth of crime rates among the young.
- Seven in ten drug users work full-time and this increases the possibility of serious accidents in the workplace.

Basic Reasons People Take Drugs

- Searching for pleasure
- Relieve pain, stress, tension, or depression
- Peer pressure
- Enhance religious or mystical experiences
- Enhance social experiences
- Enhance work performance, (i.e. amphetamine-types of drugs and cocaine)
- Drugs (primarily performance-enhancing drugs) can be used to improve athletic performance
- Relieve pain or symptoms of illness

Can you think of any additional reasons not listed above?

Notes

Nature of Addiction

Should addiction be considered:
- A bad habit?
- A failure of healthy choices?
- A failure of morality?
- A symptom of other problems?
- A chronic disease?

Costs of Addiction

- As a *major* social problem, the public's view of drug abuse and addiction has been debatable over the past 20 years while the social costs of addiction have not.
- The total criminal justice, health insurance, and other costs in the United States are roughly estimated at $90 to $185 billion annually.

Major Factors Affecting Alcohol and Drug Use

- Body size: smaller or thinner persons experience the effects of drugs more intensely
- Gender: physical make-up of women have reduced tolerance to drugs in comparison to men
- Other drugs (poly drug use): taking multiple drugs can dramatically increase drug impairment
- Fatigue or illness: increases drug effects
- Empty stomach: increases drug effects
- Strength (alcohol proof) and how the amount of the drug affects one's reaction
- Mindset: uncontrollable or impulse drinking and/or use of drugs dramatically increases drug effects

Notes

Defining Addiction

- The term **addiction** is derived from the Latin verb *addicere*, which refers to the process of binding to things. Today, the word largely refers to a chronic adherence (attachment) to drugs.
- Originally, the World Health Organization (WHO) defined it as "a state of periodic or chronic intoxication detrimental to the individual and society, which is characterized by an overwhelming desire to continue taking the drug and to obtain it by any means" (1964, pp. 9–10).
- Addiction is a complex disease.

Another Definition of Addiction

- The National Institute on Drug Abuse (NIDA) defines addiction as ". . . a chronic, relapsing brain disease that is characterized by compulsive drug-seeking and use, despite harmful consequences. It is considered a brain disease because drugs change the brain—they change its structure and how it works. These brain changes can be long lasting and can lead to the harmful behaviors seen in people who abuse drugs" (NIDA 2008a, p. 5).

The *Diagnostic and Statistical Manual of Mental Disorders*, fifth edition (DSM-5) (APA 2013)

- DSM-5 combines *substance abuse* and *substance dependence* into a single condition called ***substance use disorder***.
- The diagnosis of substance use disorder includes the following:
  - *Pharmacological* – taking the substance in larger doses
  - *Excessive time spent obtaining the substance*
  - *Craving the drug*

The *Diagnostic and Statistical Manual of Mental Disorders*, fifth edition (DSM-5) (APA 2013) (cont'd)

- *Social impairment*: failure to meet goals and obligations
- *Risky use of the substance*: despite physical and/or psychological problems encountered
- *Tolerance*: The individual needs increased amounts to achieve the diminishing effects of the drug
- *Withdrawal*: Symptoms that can often leading to renewed substance dependence

Addiction Includes Physical <u>and</u> Psychological Dependence

- **Physical dependence** refers to the body's need to constantly have the drug or drugs.
- **Psychological dependence** refers to the mental inability to stop using the drug or drugs.

Major Models of Addiction

- **Moral Model:** Poor morals and lifestyle; a choice
- **Disease Model:** A belief that addiction is both chronic and progressive, and that the drug user does not have control over the use and abuse of the drug
- **Characterological or Personality Predisposition Model:** Personality disorder, problems with the *personality* of the addicted (needs, motives, attitudes of the individual, and impulse control disorders)

Notes

Notes

Career Pattern of Addiction

- Experimentation or initiation of drug use
- Escalation: increasing use
- Maintenance: optimistic belief that the drug fits in well with day-to-day goals and activities
- Dysfunction: problems with use interfering with day-to-day goals
- Recovery: getting out of drug use/abuse
- Ex-addict: successfully quitting

Major Risk Factors for Addiction

- Alcohol and/or other drugs used alone
- Alcohol and/or other drugs used in order to reduce stress and/or anxiety
- Availability of drugs
- Abusive and/or neglectful parents; other dysfunctional family patterns
- Misperception of peer norms regarding the extent of alcohol and/or drug use (belief that many other people are using drugs)
- Alienation factors, like isolation and emptiness

Major Risk Factors for *Adolescents*

- Physical or sexual abuse (past and/or present)
- Peer norms favoring drug use
- Misperception and/or power of age group peer norms
- Conflicts, such as dependence versus independence, adult maturational tasks versus fear, and low self-esteem.

Major Risk Factors for *Adolescents* (continued)

- Teenage risk-taking and view of being omnipotent and invulnerable to drug effects
- Drug use viewed as a rite of passage into adulthood
- Drug use perceived as glamorous, fun, facilitating, and intimate
- Electronic social media influences like photos of drinking posted on MySpace

Major Risk Factors for *Adults*

- Loss of meaningful role or occupational identity due to pending retirement
- Loss, grief, or isolation due to divorce, loss of parents, or departure of children ("empty nest syndrome")
- Loss of positive body image
- Dealing with a newly diagnosed illness (e.g., diabetes, heart problems, arthritis, cancer)
- Disappointment when life's expectations are clearly not met

Biological Explanations for the Use and Abuse of Drugs

- **Biological: Genetic and biophysiological theories**
  - Addiction is based on genes, brain dysfunction, and biochemical patterns
  - Biological explanations emphasize the effects of drugs on the central nervous system (CNS)
- **Reward centers in some people are more sensitive to drugs, resulting in more pleasure and greater rewarding experiences from the use of drugs**
  - Drugs interfere with functioning neurotransmitters (neurotransmitters are chemical messengers used for communication between brain regions)

Notes

Notes

Three Principle Biological Theories

- **Abused Drugs are Positive Reinforcers**
  - Most drugs with abuse potential enhance pleasure centers by causing the release of specific brain neurotransmitters such as dopamine
- **Drug Abuse and Psychiatric Disorders**
  - Biological explanations are thought to be responsible for the substantial overlap that exists between drug addiction and mental illness
- **Genetic Explanations**
  - Inherited traits can predispose some individuals to drug addiction.

Abused Drugs as Positive Reinforcers

This explanation believes that most drugs with abuse potential *enhance the pleasure centers* by causing the release of ***dopamine***, which is a specific brain neurotransmitter.

Genetic Explanations for Contribution to Drug Abuse Vulnerability

- Character traits, such as insecurity and vulnerability, which is often found in many drug users/abusers may be genetically determined.
- Factors that determine how difficult it will be to break a drug addiction may be genetically determined.

Genetic Factors Contribute to Drug Abuse Vulnerability

- Psychiatric disorders may be relieved by taking drugs of abuse, thus encouraging their use.
- Drug users may have reward centers in the brain that may be especially sensitive to addictive drugs.
- Addiction is a medical condition in the brain of addicts.
- Addiction is genetically determined, and people with this predisposition are less likely to abandon their drug of abuse.

Psychological Explanations for Drug Use/Abuse

- Psychological theories regarding drug use and addiction mostly focus on mental or emotional states of drug users, the possible existence of unconscious motivations that are within all of us, and social and environmental factors.
- The American Psychiatric Association classifies severe drug dependence as a form of psychiatric disorder.
- Drugs that are abused can cause mental conditions that mimic major psychiatric illness.

Psychological Explanations for Drug Use/Abuse (continued)

- Psychological factors of addiction include:
  - Escape from reality
  - Boredom
  - Inability to cope with anxiety
  - Destructive self-indulgence (constantly desiring intoxicants)
  - Blind compliance with drug-abusing peers
  - Self-destructiveness
  - Blindly using drugs without wanting to understand the harmful effects of drug use
  - Self medicating (need the drug to feel better)

Notes

Notes

Theories Based on Learning

Humans acquire drug use behavior by the close association or pairing of one significant reinforcing stimulus (like friendship and intimacy) with another less significant or neutral stimulus (e.g., initial use of alcohol, marijuana, ecstasy, cocaine). In *learning* to use drugs the following occurs:

- **Conditioning:** The close association of significant reinforcing stimulus with another less significant or neutral stimulus
- **Habituation:** Repeating certain patterns of behavior until they become established or habitual
- **"Addiction to pleasure" theory:** Assumes it is biologically normal to continue a pleasure stimulus when once begun

Who Is at Risk?

- People who are at a high risk for drug use and addiction are often known as **drug sensation-seeking individuals** or simply, **sensation-seekers**.
  - Sensation-seekers continually search for new or novel thrills in their experiences, and are known to have a relentless desire to pursue physical and psychological stimulation often involving dangerous behavior.
  - Sensation-seekers attracted to drug are more likely to maintain a constant preoccupation with altering their consciousness (getting high).

Social Psychological Learning Theories

If the effects of drug use become personally rewarding, "or become reinforcing through conditioning, the chances of continuing to use are greater than stopping" (Akers 1992, p. 86).

Primary conditions determining drug use are:

- Amount of exposure to drug-using peers
- Extent of drug use in a given neighborhood
- Age of first use (exposure to drugs at younger ages results in greater difficulty in stopping drug use)
- Frequency of drug use among peers

Sociological Explanations

- **Social Influence Theories:** Focus on *microscopic* explanations that concentrate on the roles played by significant others and their impact on the individual.
- **Structural Influence Theories:** Focus on *macroscopic* explanations of drug use and the assumption that the organizational structure of society has a major impact on individual drug use.

Social Influence Theories

- **Social learning theory** explains drug use as a form of learned behavior.
- **Social influence and the role of significant others** says the use of drugs is learned during intimate interaction with others who, while using the drug, serve as a primary group.

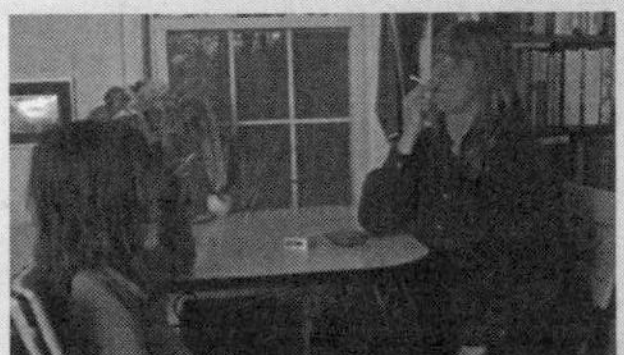

This child is role playing largely by imitating the habits of a significant other.

Social Influence Theories (continued)

- **Labeling theory** says people whose opinions we value have a determining influence over our self-image. Key factors in labeling theory include:
  - Primary deviance
  - Secondary deviance
  - Master status
  - Retrospective interpretation
  - *Can you define these four key factors used in labeling theory?*
- **Subculture theory** explains that peer pressure is a determining cause of drug experimentation, use, and/or abuse.

Notes

Notes

Structural Influence Theories

- **Structural Influence Theories:** Focus on how the *organization* of a society, group, or subculture is largely responsible for drug abuse by its members
- **Social Disorganization and Social Strain Theories:** Drug use is caused by rapid and disruptive social change in society
- **Control Theories:** Belief that if people are left without attachments (bonds) to other groups (family, peers, social institutions), they have a tendency to deviate from expected cultural values, norms, and attitudes and use drugs
  - Socialization: Internal and external controls

Danger Signals of Drug Abuse

- Do those close to you often ask about your drug use? Have they noticed changes in your moods or behavior?
- Are you defensive if a friend or relative mentions your drug or alcohol use?
- Are you sometimes embarrassed or frightened by your behavior under the influence of drugs or alcohol?

Danger Signals of Drug Abuse (continued)

- Have you ever gone to see a new doctor because your regular physician would not prescribe the drug you wanted?
- When you are under pressure or feel anxious, do you automatically take a depressant, stimulant, or drink?
- Do you take drugs more often or for purposes other than those recommended by your doctor?

Danger Signals of Drug Abuse (continued)

- Do you mix other types of drugs with alcohol?
- Do you drink or take drugs *regularly* to help you sleep?
- Do you have to take drugs to relieve boredom or get through the day?
- Do you personally think you may have a drug problem?
- Do you avoid people who do not use drugs?
- Do you believe you cannot have fun without alcohol or other drugs?

Low-Risk and High-Risk Drug Choices

- **Low-risk drug choices** refer to values and attitudes that lead to controlling the use of alcohol or drugs—self-monitoring your drug use, behavior, and abstinence.
- **High-risk drug choices** refer to developing values and attitudes that lead to using drugs both habitually and addictively, such as constantly searching for drinking and drug parties and hanging with drug abusers.

Notes

CHAPTER 3

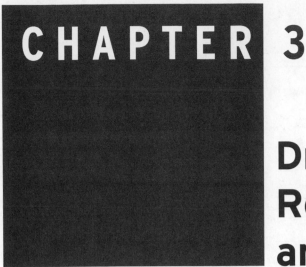

Drug Use, Regulation, and the Law

The chapter outline provides you with an organizational guide to the topics and ideas presented in this chapter of the text.

Introduction
Cultural Attitudes About Drug Use
The Road to Regulation and the FDA
- The Rising Demand for Effectiveness in Medicinal Drugs
- Regulating the Development of New Drugs
- The Effects of the OTC Review on Today's Medications

The Regulation of Drug Advertising
- Federal Regulation and Quality Assurance

Drug Abuse and the Law
- Drug Laws and Deterrence
- Factors in Controlling Drug Abuse

Strategies for Preventing Drug Abuse
- Supply Reduction Strategy
- Demand Reduction Strategy
- Inoculation Strategy
- Drug Courts

Current and Future Drug Use
- Drug Legalization Debate
- Drug Testing
- Pragmatic Drug Policies

Key Terms

Define the following terms:

1. **Thalidomide** ____________________
2. **Phocomelia** ____________________
3. **Switching policy** ____________________
4. **Supply reduction** ____________________
5. **Interdiction** ____________________
6. **Inoculation** ____________________
7. **Drug courts** ____________________
8. **Demand reduction** ____________________
9. **Harrison Act of 1914** ____________________
10. **Secure and Responsible Drug Disposal Act** ____________________

Fill-in-the-Blank

1. The ________________________________ required manufacturers to indicate the amounts of alcohol, morphine, opium, cocaine, heroin, and marijuana extract on the label of each product.
2. ________________________ is a birth defect that involves impaired development of the arms, legs, or both.
3. The first legitimate effort by the U.S. government to regulate addicting substances was the ________ ________________________________.
4. The ________________________________ allows drug companies to receive tax advantages if they develop drugs that are not very profitable.
5. ________________________________ involves attempts to decrease individuals' tendencies to use drugs with emphasis on reformulating values and behaviors.
6. The policy of cutting off or destroying supplies of illicit drugs is called ________________ ________________.

Identify

1. Identify society's two major guidelines for controlling drug development and marketing.

   a. ________________________________

   b. ________________________________

2. The Durham-Humphrey Amendment to the Food, Drug, and Cosmetic Act established criteria for determining whether a drug should be classified as prescription or nonprescription. Identify the three categories that determine whether a drug is considered nonprescription.

   a. ________________________________

   b. ________________________________

   c. ________________________________

3. Identify and explain the regulatory steps for developing new prescription drugs.

   a. ________________________________

   b. ________________________________

   c. ________________________________

4. Identify the criteria that must be satisfied if a drug is to be switched to OTC status.

a. ____________________

b. ____________________

c. ____________________

■ Discussion Questions

1. Name and explain an example of a law or an amendment that has been passed to allow an exception to FDA new prescription drug regulations. Explain why the regulation is important. ____________________

2. Discuss the effects of advertising on the drug industry. ____________________

3. Why are drug laws not always a satisfactory deterrent against the use of illicit drugs? ____________________

4. Discuss the drug legalization debate. What are the arguments being presented for and against the legalization of drugs? What are some possible compromises? What do you think is the best option?

5. Discuss the pros and cons of drug testing. ____________________

Notes

Drug Use, Regulation, and the Law

Chapter 3

Guidelines for Controlling Drug Development and Marketing

- Society has the right to protect itself from the damaging impact of drug use.
- Society has the right to demand safe and effective drugs.

Patent Medicines

- The term **patent medicines** signified that the ingredients were secret, not patented.
- The patent medicines of the late 1800s and early 1900s demonstrated the problems of insufficient regulation of the drug industry.

The 1906 Pure Food and Drug Act

- Required manufacturers to include on labels the amounts of alcohol, morphine, opium, cocaine, heroin, or marijuana extract in each product
- Did not prohibit distribution of dangerous preparations

The Sherley Amendment in 1912

- Accuracy of manufacturers' therapeutic claims was not controlled by the Pure Food and Drug Act.
- The Sherley Amendment in 1912 was passed to strengthen existing laws and required that labels should not contain "any statement ... regarding the curative or therapeutic effect ... which is false and fraudulent."

Food, Drug, and Cosmetic Act

- The sale and use of Elixir Sulfanilamide led to a tragic accident that killed over 100 people.
- Companies required to file applications with the government showing that new drugs were safe.

Notes

Notes

Food, Drug, and Cosmetic Act (continued)

- Required safe tolerances be set for unavoidable poisonous substances.
- Authorized establishment of identity and quality for foods.

Durham-Humphrey Amendment

- Made formal distinction between prescription and nonprescription drugs
- Established drug classification categories:
  - Drug is habit-forming
  - Drug is not safe for self-medication
  - Drug is a new drug and not shown to be completely safe

Kefauver-Harris Amendments

- Passed, in part, as a consequence of the thalidomide tragedy
- Drug manufacturers had to demonstrate the efficacy and safety of drugs
- The FDA was empowered to withdraw approval of a drug that was already being marketed
- The FDA was permitted to regulate and evaluate drug testing by pharmaceutical companies

Regulating New Drug Development

- The amended Food, Drug, and Cosmetic Act requires that all new drugs be registered with and approved by the FDA.

Regulating New Drug Development (continued)

- The FDA is mandated by Congress to:
  - Ensure the rights and safety of human subjects during clinical testing
  - Evaluate the safety and efficacy of new treatments
  - Compare benefits and risks of new drugs and determine if approval for marketing is appropriate

Regulatory Steps for New Prescription Drugs

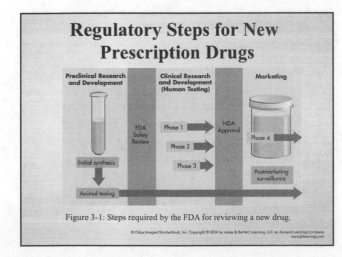

Figure 3-1: Steps required by the FDA for reviewing a new drug.

Notes

Notes

Regulatory Steps for New Prescription Drugs (continued)

- **Step 1:** Preclinical research and development
- **Step 2:** Clinical research and development
  - Initial clinical stage
  - Clinical pharmacological evaluation stage
  - Extended clinical evaluation
- **Step 3:** Permission to market
  - Postmarketing surveillance

New Drug Application (NDA)

- If there is sufficient data to demonstrate that a drug is safe and effective, the company submits an NDA as a formal request that the FDA approve it for marketing.

Exceptions: Special Drug-Marketing Laws

- "Fast-track" rule
  - Applied to testing of certain drugs, such as ones for rare cancers and AIDS
- Orphan Drug Law
  - Tax advantages for development of drugs to treat "rare diseases" since this can be otherwise unprofitable
- Prescription Drug User Fee Act of 1992
  - Increase reviewers and decrease review time

Secure and Responsible Drug Disposal Act

- Addresses the problem that patients were not allowed to return drugs to DEA registrants

The Regulation of Nonprescription Drugs

- In 1972, the FDA initiated a program to evaluate the effectiveness and safety of nonprescription drugs.
- The FDA evaluated each active ingredient in OTC medications and placed ingredients into three categories:
  - I. Generally recognized as safe and effective
  - II. Not safe and effective or unacceptable indications
  - III. Insufficient data to permit final classification

Switching Policy

- The drug must have been used by prescription for 3 years.
- Use must have been relatively high during the time it was used by prescription.
- Adverse drug reactions must not be alarming, and the frequency of side effects must not have increased during the time the drug was available to the public.

Notes

Notes

Drug Advertising

- Promotional efforts by pharmaceutical companies have a large impact on the drug-purchasing habits of the general public and health professionals.
- As a general rule, the FDA oversees most issues related to advertising of prescription products. The FTC regulates OTC advertising.

Direct-to-Consumer (DTC) Advertising

- Most physicians surveyed agreed that because their patient saw a DTC advertisement, he/she asked thoughtful questions during the visit. Approximately the same percentage of physicians thought the advertisements made their patients more aware of possible treatments.
- The physicians surveyed indicated that the advertisements did not convey information about risks and benefits equally well.

Direct-to-Consumer (DTC) Advertising (continued)

- Approximately 75% of physicians surveyed indicated that DTC ads cause patients to think that the drug works better than it does, and many physicians felt some pressure to prescribe something when patients mentioned DTC ads.
- The physicians surveyed reported that patients understand that they need to consult a health care provider concerning appropriate treatments.

The Harrison Act of 1914

- Marked the first legitimate effort by the federal government to regulate and control the production and importation of addicting substances

The Comprehensive Drug Abuse Prevention and Control Act

- This 1970 act divided substances with abuse potential into categories based on the degree of their abuse potential and clinical usefulness.
- Schedules I, II, III, IV, and V

"Scheduling"

- **Schedule I** substances have high-abuse potential and no currently approved medicinal uses.
- **Schedule II** substances have high-abuse potential but are approved for medical uses and can be prescribed.
- **Schedule II–V** substances reflect the likelihood of abuse and clinical usefulness.

Notes

Notes

Factors Determining Scheduling

- The actual or relative potential for abuse of the drug.
- Scientific evidence of the pharmacological effects of the drug.
- The state of current scientific knowledge regarding the substance.
- Its history and current pattern of abuse.
- What, if any, risk there is to the public health.

Factors Determining Scheduling (continued)

- The psychological or physiological dependence liability of the drug.
- The scope, duration, and significance of abuse.
- Whether the substance is an immediate precursor of a substance already controlled.

Principal Issues Influencing Laws Regarding Substance Abuse

- If a person abuses a drug, should he or she be treated as a criminal or as a sick person inflicted with a disease?
- How is the user (supposedly the victim) distinguished from the pusher (supposedly the criminal) of an illicit drug, and who should be more harshly punished?
- Are the laws and associated penalties effective deterrents against drug use or abuse, and how is effectiveness determined?

Strategies for Preventing Drug Abuse

- **Supply Reduction**
  - Attempts to curtail the supply of illegal drugs or their precursors and exert greater control over other, more therapeutic drugs
  - Includes interdiction, the policy of cutting off or destroying supplies of illicit drugs
  - Limited success

Strategies for Preventing Drug Abuse (continued)

- **Inoculation**
  - Aims to protect drug users by teaching them responsibility and explaining the effects of drugs on bodily and mental functioning
- **Demand Reduction**
  - Aims to reduce the actual demand for drugs

Suggestions for Reducing Demand

- A top priority of prevention is to reduce demand by youth.
- Education must be carefully designed for the target population.
- Attitudes toward drug abuse must be changed.
- Replacement therapy can be useful.

Notes

Notes

Drug Courts

- Designed to deal with nonviolent, drug-abusing offenders
- Integrate mandatory drug testing, substance abuse treatment, sanctions, and incentives in a judicially supervised setting

Drug Legalization Debate

- Violence and crime would decrease/increase?
- Profits associated with illegal trade would decrease/increase?
- Law enforcement costs would decrease/increase?
- Addiction would decrease/increase?
- Societal/health costs would decrease/increase?
- Consumption would increase/decrease?

© Odua Images/ShutterStock, Inc. Copyright © 2014 by Jones & Bartlett Learning, LLC an Ascend Learning Company www.jblearning.com

Drug Testing

- In response to the demand by society to stop the spread of drug abuse and its adverse consequences, drug testing has been implemented in some situations to detect drug users.
  - Breathalyzers
  - Urine, blood, and hair specimens

© Odua Images/ShutterStock, Inc. Copyright © 2014 by Jones & Bartlett Learning, LLC an Ascend Learning Company www.jblearning.com

Pragmatic Drug Policies

- The government must develop programs that are consistent with the desires of the majority of the population.
- Programs must consider de-emphasizing interdiction and stress programs that reduce demand.

Pragmatic Drug Policies (continued)

- Government and society must better understand how laws, used properly and selectively, can reinforce and communicate expected social behavior and values.
- Programs, such as anti-smoking campaigns, should be implemented that employ "public consensus" more effectively.

Notes

CHAPTER 4

Homeostatic Systems and Drugs

The chapter outline provides you with an organizational guide to the topics and ideas presented in this chapter of the text.

Key Terms

Define the following terms:

1. **Homeostasis** ______
2. **Hormones** ______
3. **Neurons** ______
4. **Glia** ______
5. **Axons** ______
6. **Receptors** ______
7. **Psychoactive** ______
8. **Genetics** ______
9. **Molecular biology** ______
10. **Synapse** ______
11. **Dendrites** ______
12. **Opiate receptors** ______

13. **Endorphins** ______________________________

14. **Cannabinoid** ______________________________

15. **Anandamide** ______________________________

16. **Agonistic** ______________________________

17. **Nicotinic** ______________________________

18. **Muscarinic** ______________________________

19. **Sympathomimetics** ______________________________

20. **Nucleus accumbens** ______________________________

21. **Hormones** ______________________________

22. **Anabolic steroids** ______________________________

23. **Androgens** ______________________________

24. **Neurotransmitters** ______________________________

■ Fill-in-the-Blank

1. Chemical messengers released by neurons are called ______________________.

2. Drugs that affect mood or alter the state of consciousness are called ______________________ ______________________.

3. ______________________ are chemical messengers released into the blood by glands.

4. A ______________________ is a minute gap between a neuron and target cell, across which neurotransmitters travel.

5. ______________________ are short branches of neurons that receive transmitter signals.

6. Receptors activated by opioid narcotic drugs such as heroin and morphine are called ______________________ ______________________.

7. Receptors activated by THC in marijuana are called ______________________.

8. A drug may have two different effects on a receptor when interaction occurs: ______________________ __________ or ______________________.

9. Agents that mimic the effects of norepinephrine or epinephrine are ______________________ __________.

10. Male sex hormones are called ______________________.

11. The natural neurotransmitter that activates cannabinoid receptors is ______________________.

12. There are two main types of cells in the brain, one type is the neuron, the other is the ______________________.

Identify

1. Identify and describe three neurotransmitters.

a. ______________________________

b. ______________________________

c. ______________________________

2. Identify three brain regions that are influenced by drugs of abuse and describe characteristics of each.

a. ______________________________

____

b. ______________________________

____

c. ______________________________

____

Discussion Questions

1. Describe the process of sending messages by neurons. ______________________________

____

____

____

2. Why are many athletes (and some nonathletes) attracted to androgens? What are the hormones' positive and negative side effects? Do you think that classifying anabolic steroids as Schedule III drugs is justified?

____

____

____

3. How could damage to the frontal cortex of the brain be associated with drug abuse? ______________________________

____

____

____

4. Describe the difference between an agonist and an antagonist drug. ______________________________

____

____

____

Notes

Homeostatic Systems and Drugs

Chapter 4

Homeostasis

Internal and external changes in the environment

↓

Body self-regulates via nervous system and endocrine system

↓

Equilibrium

Introduction to Nervous Systems

- All nervous systems consist of specialized nerve cells called *neurons* and *glia* (supporting cells).
- Neurons are responsible for conducting the homeostatic functions of the brain and other parts of the nervous system by receiving and sending information.
- Sending and receiving information is an electrochemical process.

Transfer of Messages by Neurons

- The receiving region of the neuron is affected by a chemical message that either excites or inhibits it.
- Neuronal message:
  - Impulse moves from the receiving region of the neuron down the axon to the sending region (*terminal*).
  - Chemical messengers (*neurotransmitters*) are released.

Transfer of Messages by Neurons (continued)

- Neurotransmitters travel and attach to receiving proteins called *receptors* on target cells.
- Activation of receptors causes a change in the activity of the target cell; the target cells can be other neurons or cells that make up organs, muscles, or glands.

Sending Messages by Neurons

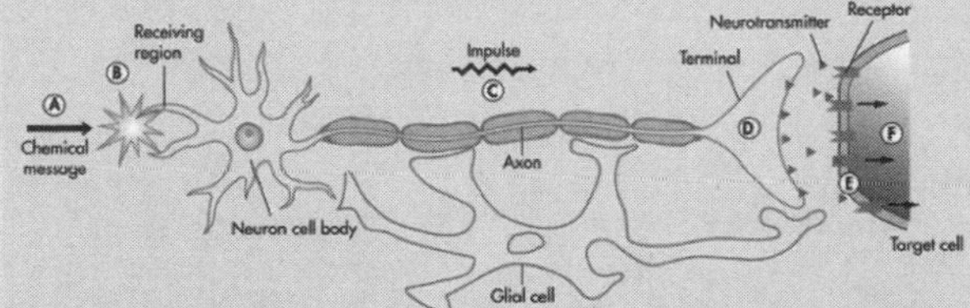

Figure 4-1: The process of sending messages by neurons. The receiving region (B) of the neuron is activated by an incoming message (A) near the neuronal cell body. The neuron sends an electricity-like chemical impulse (C) down the axon to its terminal (D). The impulse causes the release of neurotransmitters from the terminal to transmit the message to the target. This is done when the neurotransmitter molecules activate the receptors on the membranes of the target cell (E). The activated receptors then cause a change to occur in intracellular functions of the target cell (F). Glial cells (glia) surround the neurons and their axons as insulation to enhance their abilities to send impulses and to support their other cellular functions.

Notes

Notes

Neurons and Neurotransmitters

- Neurons can send discrete excitatory or inhibitory messages to their target cells.
- Neurons are distinguished by the type of neurotransmitter they release.
- Neurotransmitters represent a wide variety of chemical substances and functions.
  - Example: Dopamine activates the pleasure center.

Common Neurotransmitters

Neurotransmitter	Type of Effect	CNS Changes	Drugs of Abuse
Dopamine	Inhibitory-excitatory	Euphoria Agitation Paranoia Altered	Amphetamines, Cocaine "Bath salts" active ingredients
GABA	Inhibitory	Cognition Sedation Relaxation Drowsiness Depression	Alcohol, valium-type barbiturates

Common Neurotransmitters (continued)

Serotonin	Inhibitory	Sleep Relaxation Sedation	LSD
Acetylcholine	Excitatory-inhibitory	Mild euphoria Excitation Insomnia	Tobacco, nicotine
Endorphins	Inhibitory	Mild euphoria Block pain	Narcotics

Common Neurotransmitters (continued)

Anandamide	Inhibitory	Relaxation Increase sense of well-being	Tetrahydro-cannabinol (marijuana-like) "spice" active ingredient

Neurons

- **Dendrites** are the receiving regions of a neuron's cell body.
- Each neuron in the central nervous system is in close proximity with other neurons.
- Although they are close, neurons never actually touch.
- **Synapse** is the point of communication between one neuron and another.
- **Synaptic cleft** is the gap between neurons at the synapse.

Neurons (continued)

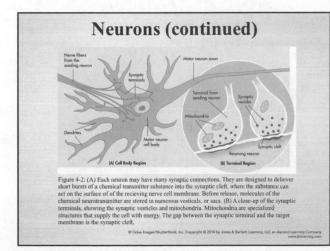

Figure 4-2: (A) Each neuron may have many synaptic connections. They are designed to deliever short bursts of a chemical transmitter substance into the synaptic cleft, where the substance can act on the surface of of the recieving nerve cell membrane. Before release, molecules of the chemical neurotransmitter are stored in numerous vesticals, or sacs. (B) A close-up of the synaptic terminals, showing the synaptic vesticles and mitochondria. Mitochondria are specialized structures that supply the cell with energy. The gap between the synaptic terminal and the target membrane is the synaptic cleft.

Notes

Notes

Synapses

- **Excitatory synapse** initiates an impulse in the receiving neuron when stimulated, causing release of neurotransmitters or increasing activity in target cell.
- **Inhibitory synapse** diminishes likelihood of an impulse in the receiving neuron or reduces the activity in other target cells.

Synapses (continued)

- A receiving neuron or target cell may have many synapses.
- Final cellular activity is a *summation* of these many excitatory and inhibitory synaptic signals.

Drug Receptors

- The chemical messengers from glands and neurons exert their effects by interacting with special protein regions in membranes called *receptors*.
- Receptors only interact with molecules that have specific configurations.

Drug Receptors (continued)

Extracellular (outside the cell)
Receptor protein (activated by neurotransmitter)
Phospholipid bilayer
Water-soluble layer
Fat-soluble layer
Water-soluble layer
Intracellular (inside the cell)

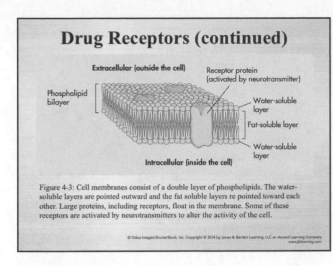

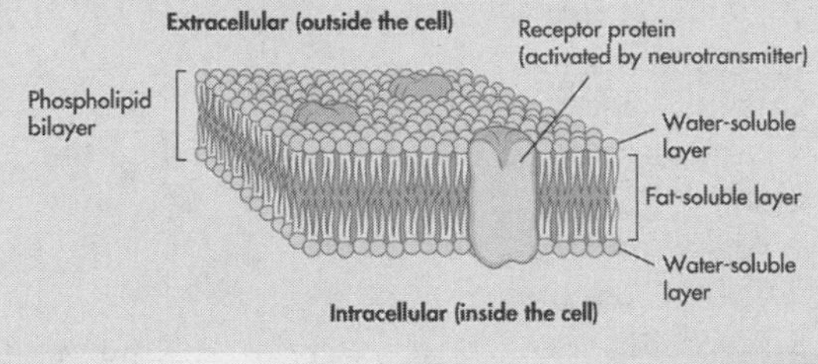

Figure 4-3: Cell membranes consist of a double layer of phospholipids. The water-soluble layers are pointed outward and the fat soluble layers re pointed toward each other. Large proteins, including receptors, float in the membrane. Some of these receptors are activated by neurotransmitters to alter the activity of the cell.

Drug Receptors (continued)

- **Agonists:** Substances or drugs that activate receptors
- **Antagonists:** Substances or drugs that attach to receptors and prevent them from being activated

Drug Receptors (continued)

Agonist (fits with and activates a receptor)
Antagonist (can occupy receptor but does not activate it)
Receptors
Cell membrane
Activation of the receptor causes a cellular function to be increased or decreased

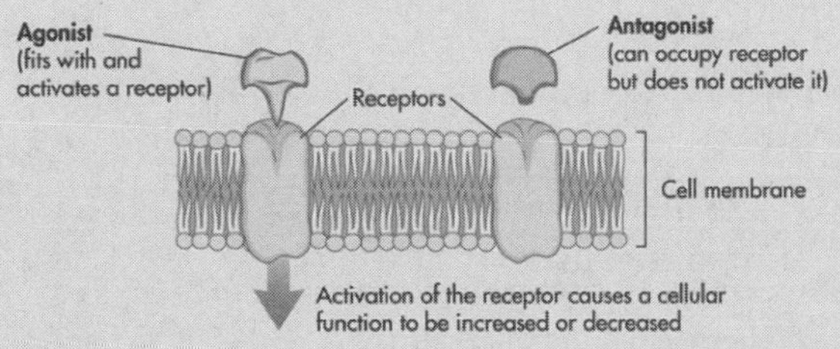

Figure 4-4: Interaction of agonist and antagonist with membrane receptor. When this receptor is occupied and activated by an agonist, it can cause cellular changes.

Notes

Notes

Neurotransmitters

- Many drugs affect the activity of neurotransmitters by altering their synthesis, storage, release, or deactivation.
- Neurotransmitters frequently altered by drugs of abuse:
  - Acetylcholine
  - Catecholamines
  - Serotonin
  - GABA
  - Endorphins
  - Anandamide

Tyrosine

L-DOPA

Dopamine

Norepinephrine

Epinephrine

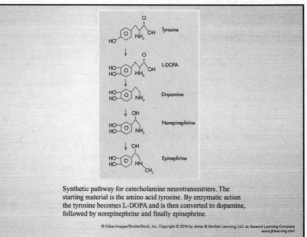

Synthetic pathway for catecholamine neurotransmitters. The starting material is the amino acid tyrosine. By enzymatic action the tyrosine becomes L-DOPA and is then converted to dopamine, followed by norepinephrine and finally epinephrine.

Major Divisions of the Nervous System

- Two major components of the nervous system
  - Central nervous system (CNS)
  - Peripheral nervous system (PNS)

Central Nervous System

- CNS includes the brain and the spinal cord
- CNS receives information from PNS, evaluates the information, then regulates muscle and organ activity via PNS Reticular activating system
  - Receives input from all the sensory systems and cerebral cortex
  - Controls the brain's state of arousal (sleep vs. awake)
  - Reticular activating system

Central Nervous System (continued)

- Basal ganglia
  - Controls motor activity
  - Establishes and maintains behaviors
- Limbic system
  - Regulates emotional activities, memory, reward, and endocrine activity
  - Includes the nucleus accumbens, the brain's reward center
  - Dopamine

Central Nervous System (continued)

- The cerebral cortex
  - Helps interpret, process, and respond to information; selects appropriate behavior and suppresses inappropriate behavior
- The hypothalamus
  - Controls endocrine and basic body functions

Notes

Notes

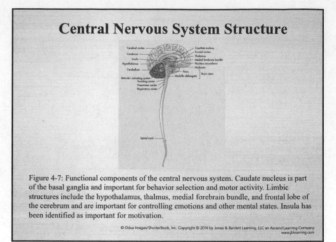

Central Nervous System Structure

Figure 4-7: Functional components of the central nervous system. Caudate nucleus is part of the basal ganglia and important for behavior selection and motor activity. Limbic structures include the hypothalamus, thalmus, medial forebrain bundle, and frontal lobe of the cerebrum and are important for controlling emotions and other mental states. Insula has been identified as important for motivation.

Peripheral Nervous System

- Consists of input and output nerves
- **Input** to brain and spinal cord
  - Conveys sensory info (pain, pressure, temperature)
- **Output:** Two types
  - Somatic (control of voluntary muscles)
  - Autonomic (control of unconscious functions)

Autonomic Nervous System

- Sympathetic and parasympathetic system
  - These systems work in an antagonistic fashion to control unconscious, visceral functions such as breathing and cardiovascular activity
- Sympathetic system
  - Norepinephrine
- Parasympathetic system
  - Acetylcholine

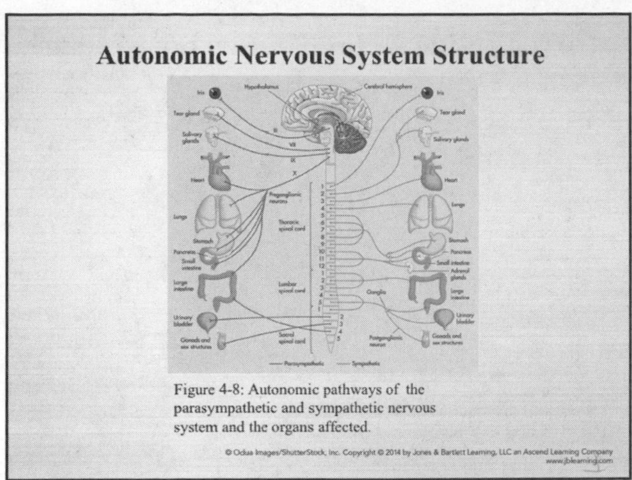
Autonomic Nervous System Structure
Figure 4-8: Autonomic pathways of the parasympathetic and sympathetic nervous system and the organs affected.
© Odua Images/ShutterStock, Inc. Copyright © 2014 by Jones & Bartlett Learning, LLC an Ascend Learning Company
www.jblearning.com

Introduction to the Endocrine System

- The endocrine system consists of secreting glands (e.g., adrenal, thyroid, pituitary)
- These glands produce substances called hormones (e.g., adrenaline, steroids, insulin, sex hormones)
- These substances are information transferring molecules

Introduction to the Endocrine System (continued)

- Hormones are secreted into the bloodstream and carried by the blood to all the organs and tissues of the body.
- Hormones affect selected tissues that are designed to receive the information.
- Hormones may be highly selective or very general with regard to the cells or organs they influence.

Notes

Notes

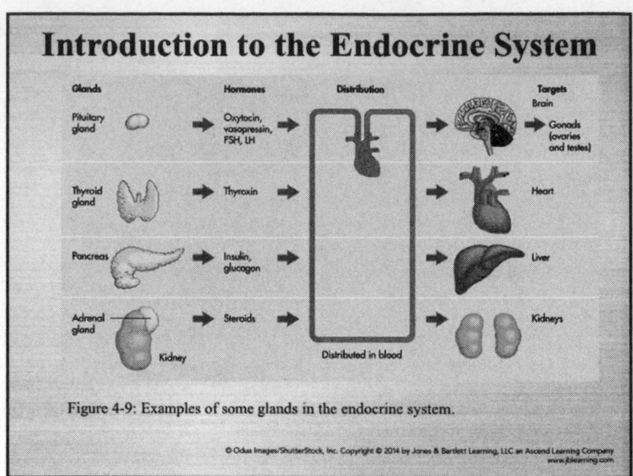

The Abuse of Hormones: Anabolic Steroids

- Androgens
  - Produce growth of muscle mass
  - Increase body weight
- Anabolic steroids
  - Are structurally related to the male hormone testosterone
  - Sometimes abused by athletes and body builders to improve strength and appearances
  - Controlled as Schedule III substances

CHAPTER 5

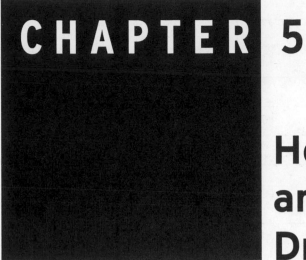

How and Why Drugs Work

The chapter outline provides you with an organizational guide to the topics and ideas presented in this chapter of the text.

Key Terms

Define the following terms:

1. **Side effects** ____________________
2. **Withdrawal** ____________________
3. **Tolerance** ____________________
4. **Synergism** ____________________
5. **Threshold dose** ____________________
6. **Blood–brain barrier** ____________________
7. **Pharmacokinetics** ____________________
8. **Half-life** ____________________

9. **Metabolism (metabolite)** ______________________________

10. **Reverse tolerance** ______________________________

11. **Dependence** ______________________________

12. **Rebound effect** ______________________________

13. **Cross-tolerance** ______________________________

14. **Mental set** ______________________________

15. **Placebo effect** ______________________________

16. **Dysphoric** ______________________________

■ Fill-in-the-Blank

1. The correlation between the amount of a drug given and its effects is ______________________.

2. ______________________ occurs when the presence of one drug alters the action of another drug.

3. The ______________________ is selective filtering between the cerebral blood vessels and the brain.

4. The use of vaccines against cocaine causes the body to produce antibodies ______________ against the drug and prevent it from passing across the ______________________.

5. The maximum drug effect, regardless of dose, is the ______________________.

6. The ______________________ is the buildup of a drug in the body after multiple doses taken at short intervals.

7. The process of changing the chemical properties of a drug, usually by metabolism, is called ______________________.

8. Chemical products of metabolism are called ______________________.

9. Something that causes physical defects in the fetus is said to have ______________________ properties.

10. Paradoxical effects that occur when a drug has been eliminated from the body are called ______________________.

11. ______________________ occurs when dependence on a drug can be relieved by other similar drugs.

■ Identify

1. Identify five pharmacokinetic issues that should be considered when attempting to anticipate a drug's effects.

a. ______

b. ______

c. ______

d. ______

e. ______

2. Identify and describe four methods of taking drugs.

a. ______

b. ______

c. ______

d. ______

3. Identify three ways an injection may be administered.

a. ______

b. ______

c. ______

4. Identify four possible side effects that can result from drug use.

a. ______

b. ______

c. ______

d. ______

5. Identify four factors that affect a drug's distribution.

a. ______

b. ______

c. ______

d. ______

■ Matching

Match the drug interaction with its description:

___ Additive interactions

___ Potentiation

___ Synergism

___ Antagonistic interactions

a. effects created when drugs cancel one another out

b. ability of one drug to enhance the effect of another

c. effects created when drugs are similar and actions are added together

Discussion Questions

1. Discuss the difference between potency and toxicity. What factors determine a drug's potency? _______

2. Why is it important for people to be aware of drug interactions? _______

3. Discuss the importance of time as a factor in the body's response to a drug. _______

4. Discuss how drug effects can be modified by factors such as age, gender, and pregnancy. Why is it important for those with diseases to be especially careful when taking drugs? _______

5. Discuss how vaccines against nicotine help to treat someone with nicotine addiction. _______

6. Explain the value of drug testing when treating drug addiction. _______

7. Discuss psychological dependence. How does it develop? What are its effects? How does psychological dependence on such things as tobacco and caffeine-containing beverages differ from dependence on other substances? _______

8. What is your mental set? What factors in your life contribute to your view of drugs? _______

9. What factors do you think most influence the risk of drug abuse for an individual? Many are mentioned in the text. Can you think of any others? _______

Notes

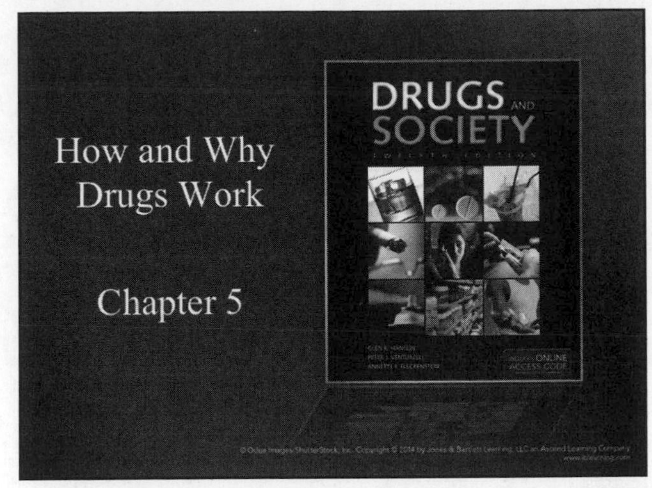
How and Why
Drugs Work
Chapter 5
DRUGS AND SOCIETY

Intended and Unintended Effects of Drugs

- Intended responses:
  - Reason for using the drug
- Unintended responses:
  - Side effects
- The main distinction between intended responses and side effects depends on the therapeutic objective.

Common Side Effects of Drugs

- Nausea or vomiting
- Changes in mental alertness
- Dependence
  - Withdrawal
- Allergic reactions
- Changes in cardiovascular activity

Notes

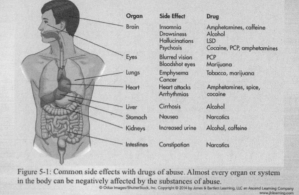

Common Side Effects of Drug

Organ	Side Effect	Drug
Brain	Insomnia	Amphetamines, caffeine
	Drowsiness	Alcohol
	Hallucinations	LSD
	Psychosis	Cocaine, PCP, amphetamines
Eyes	Blurred vision	PCP
	Bloodshot eyes	Marijuana
Lungs	Emphysema Cancer	Tobacco, marijuana
Heart	Heart attacks Arrhythmias	Amphetamines, spice, cocaine
Liver	Cirrhosis	Alcohol
Stomach	Nausea	Narcotics
Kidneys	Increased urine	Alcohol, caffeine
Intestines	Constipation	Narcotics

Figure 5-1: Common side effects with drugs of abuse. Almost every organ or system in the body can be negatively affected by the substances of abuse.

Dose-Response

- Many factors can affect the way an individual responds to a drug, including the following:
  - Dose
  - Tolerance
  - Potency

Dose-Response (continued)

- Additional factors
  - Pharmacokinetic properties:
    - Rate of absorption
    - Manner distributed throughout the body
    - Rate metabolized and eliminated
  - Form of the drug
  - Manner in which the drug is administered

Dose-Response Curve

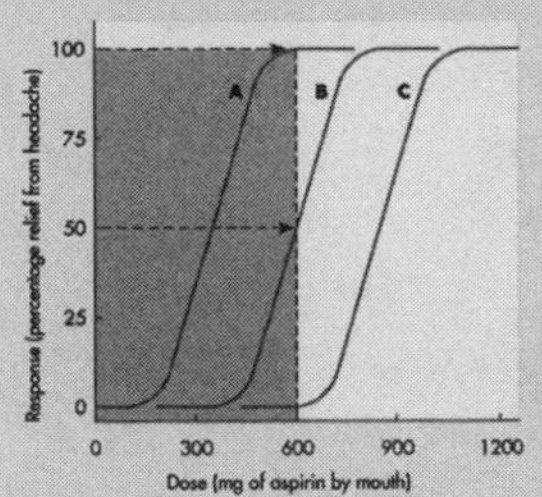

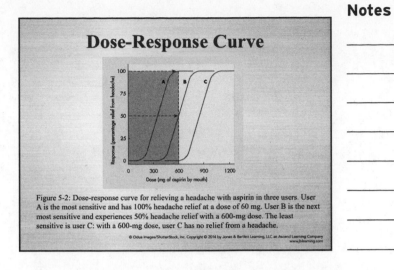

Figure 5-2: Dose-response curve for relieving a headache with aspirin in three users. User A is the most sensitive and has 100% headache relief at a dose of 60 mg. User B is the next most sensitive and experiences 50% headache relief with a 600-mg dose. The least sensitive is user C: with a 600-mg dose, user C has no relief from a headache.

Margin of Safety

- The range in dose between the amount of drug necessary to cause a therapeutic effect and a toxic effect.

Potency vs. Toxicity

- **Potency:** The amount of drug necessary to cause an effect

- **Toxicity:** The capacity of a drug to do damage or cause adverse effects in the body

Notes

Notes

Drug Interaction

- Additive effects
  - Summation of effects of drugs taken concurrently
- Antagonistic (inhibitory) effects
  - One drug cancels or blocks effects of another
- Potentiative (synergistic) effects
  - Effect of a drug is enhanced by another drug or substance

Pharmacokinetic Factors That Influence Drug Effects

- Administration
- Absorption
- Distribution
- Inactivation
- Biotransformation and elimination

Forms and Methods of Taking Drugs

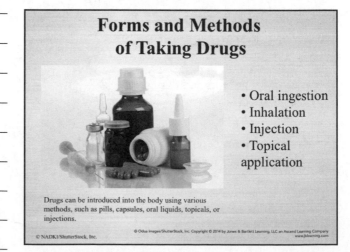

- Oral ingestion
- Inhalation
- Injection
- Topical application

Drugs can be introduced into the body using various methods, such as pills, capsules, oral liquids, topicals, or injections.

Distribution

- Most drugs are distributed throughout the body in the blood.
- It takes approximately 1 minute for a drug to circulate throughout the body after it enters the bloodstream.
- Drugs have different patterns of distribution depending on their chemical properties.

Required Doses for Effects

- **Threshold dose:** The minimum amount of a drug necessary to have an effect
- **Plateau effect:** The maximum effect a drug can have regardless of the dose
- **Cumulative effect:** The buildup of drug concentration in the body due to multiple doses taken within short intervals

Time-Response Factors

- The closer a drug is placed to the target area, the faster the onset of action.
- **Acute drug response:**
  - Immediate or short-term effects after a single drug dose
- **Chronic drug response:**
  - Long-term effects after a single dose

Notes

Notes

Biotransformation

- **Biotransformation:** The process of changing the chemical or pharmacological properties of a drug by metabolism.
- The liver is the major organ that metabolizes drugs in the body.
- The kidney is the next most important organ for drug elimination.

Physiological Variables That Modify Drug Effects

- Age
- Gender
- Pregnancy

Adaptive Processes

- **Tolerance:** Changes causing decreased response to a set dose of a drug
- **Dependence:** The physiological and psychological changes or adaptations that occur in response to the frequent administration of a drug
- **Withdrawal**

Adaptive Processes

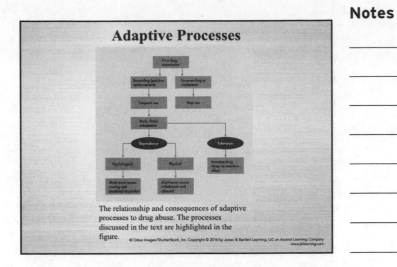

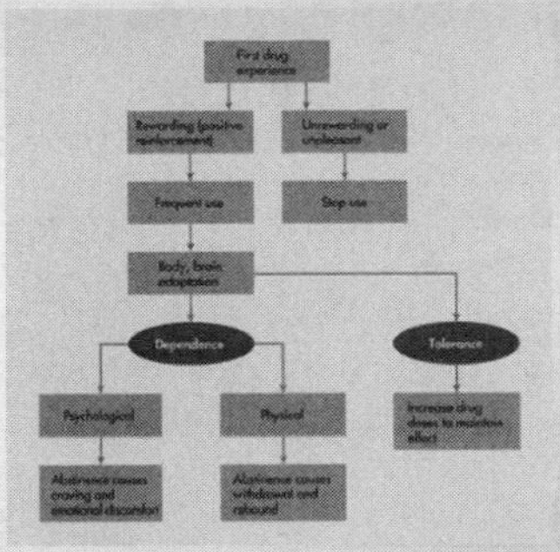

The relationship and consequences of adaptive processes to drug abuse. The processes discussed in the text are highlighted in the figure.

Tolerance

- **Reverse tolerance (sensitization):** Enhanced response to a given drug dose; opposite of tolerance
- **Cross-tolerance:** Development of tolerance to one drug causes tolerance to related drugs

Drug Dependence

Physical Dependence (e.g.,withdrawal and rebound)

Psychological Dependence (e.g., craving)

Notes

Notes

Psychological Factors Affecting Drug Effect

- Individual's mental set
- Placebo effects

Addiction and Abuse

- The use of the term *addiction* is sometimes confusing. It is often used interchangeably with dependence, either physiological or psychological in nature; other times, it is used synonymously with the term drug abuse. A more accurate definition is the compulsive drug use despite negative consequences.

Addiction and Abuse (continued)

- Factors affecting variability in dependence/addiction:
  - Hereditary factors (genetic variants); responsible for 40–60% vulnerability
  - Drug craving

Addiction and Abuse (continued)

- Other factors contributing to drug use patterns:
  - Positive versus negative effects of drug
  - Peer pressure
  - Home, school, and work environment
  - Mental state

Notes

CHAPTER 6

CNS Depressants: Sedative-Hypnotics

The chapter outline provides you with an organizational guide to the topics and ideas presented in this chapter of the text.

Key Terms

Define the following terms:

1. **Barbiturates** ______________________________
2. **Antihistamines** ______________________________
3. **Anxiolytic** ______________________________
4. **Hypnotics** ______________________________
5. **Amnesiac** ______________________________
6. **Club drug** ______________________________
7. **Paradoxical effects** ______________________________
8. **Detoxification** ______________________________

Fill-in-the-Blank

1. The most popular and safest prescription CNS depressants in use today are ______________________ ______________________.
2. ______________________ are CNS depressants used to relieve anxiety, fear, and apprehension.

3. CNS depressants used to induce drowsiness and encourage sleep are ____________________.

4. ____________________ is used to achieve a controlled state of unconsciousness so that a patient can be treated, usually by surgery, in relative comfort and without memory of an unpleasant experience.

5. The restive phase of sleep associated with dreaming is called ____________________.

6. A drug used at all-night raves, parties, dance clubs, and bars to enhance sensory experiences is called a ____________________.

7. Propofol is clinically used as a ____________________.

■ Identify

1. Why are CNS depressants problematic? Give four reasons.

   a. ____________________

   b. ____________________

   c. ____________________

   d. ____________________

2. Identify four medical uses of benzodiazepines.

   a. ____________________

   b. ____________________

   c. ____________________

   d. ____________________

3. What are some common side effects of benzodiazepines? ____________________

4. Identify three ways that benzodiazepines are abused.

   a. ____________________

   b. ____________________

   c. ____________________

5. Identify and briefly describe three other kinds of CNS depressants (CNS depressants other than barbiturates and benzodiazepines).

   a. ____________________

   b. ____________________

   c. ____________________

True/False

Tell whether each statement is true or false. If false, explain why the statement is incorrect.

1. All CNS depressants are created equal. ______________________

2. Benzodiazepines are primarily distinguished by their duration of action. ______________________

3. Antihistamines produce the same responses in all people. ______________________

4. Propofol is being abused because of its short action. ______________________

Discussion Questions

1. What is GABA? How do benzodiazepines affect GABA? ______________________

2. What are benzodiazepine receptors? ______________________

3. What are some negative effects of benzodiazepines such as Halcion and Xanax? Do you think the FDA made the right decision when it allowed Halcion to stay on the market despite court rulings and critic complaints? ______________________

4. Why are benzodiazepines preferred over barbiturates? What are the effects of uncontrolled use of barbiturates? ______________________

5. What types of people are most likely to abuse CNS depressants? What are some ways in which these people use CNS depressants? ______________________

6. What is GHB, and why is it abused? ______________________

7. How are withdrawals from CNS depressants treated? What are some of the dangers associated with treating individuals who are severely dependent on these drugs? ______________________________

____

____

____

Notes

CNS Depressants: Sedative-Hypnotics

Chapter 6

Introduction to CNS Depressants

- Why are CNS depressants problematic?
  - Usually prescribed under physician's direction
  - Second most frequently abused prescription drug and sometimes contributes to death due to accidental overdoses
  - Can cause very alarming and dangerous behavior if not closely monitored
    - Most problems associated with these drugs due to inadequate professional supervision

Introduction to CNS Depressants (continued)

- Why are CNS depressants problematic?
  - Seemingly unrelated drug groups can cause CNS depression
  - Combination use can cause dangerous drug interactions
  - Can cause disruptive personality changes

Notes

The History of CNS Depressants

- Attempts to find CNS depressants other than alcohol began in the 1800s.
- Bromides were introduced to treat nervousness and anxiety in the 1800s.
  - Very popular but toxic
- In the early 1900s, bromides were replaced by barbiturates.
  - Initially heralded as safe and effective
  - Apparent problems with tolerance, dependence, and safety

The History of CNS Depressants (continued)

- In the 1950s the first benzodiazepines were marketed as substitutes for barbiturates.
  - Relatively safe when used for short periods
  - Long-term use can cause dependence and withdrawal problems

The History of CNS Depressants (continued)

- Benzodiazepines were routinely prescribed for stress, anxiety, or apprehension.
  - In 1973, 100 million prescriptions were written for benzodiazepines.
  - Twice as many women as men taking them.
- As medical community became aware of the problem, use of depressants declined, but benzodiazepines remained still very popular.
- Classified as Schedule V drugs

The Effects of CNS Depressants

- CNS depressants reduce CNS activity and diminish the brain's level of awareness.
- Depressant drugs include:
  - Benzodiazepines
  - Barbiturate-like drugs
  - Alcohol
  - Antihistamines
  - Opioid narcotics like heroin

The Effects of CNS Depressants (continued)

- Depressants are usually classified according to the degree of their medical effects on the body. For example:
  - **Sedatives** cause mild depression and relaxation
    - *Anxiolytic*—drugs that relieve anxiety
  - **Hypnotics** induce drowsiness and encourage sleep
    - *Amnesiac* effects can cause the loss of memory

The Effects of CNS Depressants (continued)

- The same drug can cause different effects depending on dose.
  - Low dose (sedatives—relieve anxiety and promote relaxation)
  - Higher doses (hypnotics—can cause drowsiness and promote sleep)
  - Even higher doses (anesthetics can cause anesthesia and are used for patient management during surgery)

Notes

Notes

Types of CNS Depressants

- **Benzodiazepines: Valium-Type Drugs**
  - Prescribed for anxiety, relaxation and sleep
- Medical uses
  - Relief from anxiety, treatment of neurosis, relaxation of muscles, alleviation of lower-back pain, treatment of convulsive disorders, induction of sleep, relief from withdrawal symptoms, induction of amnesia

Types of CNS Depressants (continued)

- Mechanisms of action for benzodiazepine
  - Affect neurons that have receptors for the neurotransmitter GABA
- **GABA:** most common inhibitory transmitter in brain regions
  - Limbic system (alter mood)
  - RAS (cause drowsiness)
  - Motor cortex (relax muscles)

Types of CNS Depressants (continued)

- Types of benzodiazepines
  - Many benzodiazepine compounds available in the United States
  - Distinguished primarily by their duration of action: *short-acting* (hypnotics), *long-acting* (sedatives)
- Side effects include drowsiness to paradoxical effects (e.g. increased restlessness), tolerance, dependence, withdrawal, and abuse

Types of CNS Depressants (continued)

- **Barbiturates** played an important historical role as sedative-hypnotic agents.
- However, due to their narrow margin of safety and their abuse liability, they were replaced by benzodiazepines.
  - Caused many negative side effects, from nausea to death, from respiratory or cardiovascular depression

Other Types of CNS Depressants

- Drugs with barbiturate-like properties:
  - Chloral hydrate
  - Glutethimide
  - Methyprylon
  - Methaqualone
- Antihistamines
- Propofol (abused general anesthetic)
- GHB (gamma hydroxybutyrate)

Patterns of Abuse with CNS Depressants

- The American Psychiatric Association considers dependence on CNS depressants a psychiatric disorder.

Notes

Notes

Patterns of Abuse with CNS Depressants (continued)

- People most likely to abuse CNS depressants include individuals who:
  - Use drugs to relieve continual stress
  - Paradoxically feel euphoria and stimulation from depressants
  - Use depressants to counteract the unpleasant effects of other drugs of abuse
  - Combine depressants with alcohol and heroin to potentiate the effects

Patterns of Abuse with CNS Depressants (continued)

- **Detoxification:** The elimination of a toxic substance, such as a drug, and its effects
  - With CNS depressants, this is achieved by substituting a longer-acting barbiturate for the offending CNS depressant and gradually reducing the dose to avoid unpleasant withdrawal effects. Withdrawal from CNS depressants, if not managed properly, can be very dangerous, or even fatal.

CHAPTER 7

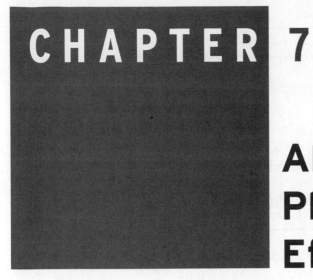

Alcohol: Pharmacological Effects

The chapter outline provides you with an organizational guide to the topics and ideas presented in this chapter of the text.

■ Key Terms

Define the following terms:

1. **Fermentation** ______________________________
2. **Distillation** ______________________________
3. **Ethanol** ______________________________
4. **Social lubricant** ______________________________
5. **Blood alcohol concentration (BAC)** ______________________________
6. **Behavioral tolerance** ______________________________
7. **Hepatotoxic effect** ______________________________

8. **Cirrhosis** ______________________________

9. **Fetal Alcohol Syndrome (FAS)** ______________________________

10. **Alcoholic cardiomyopathy** ______________________________

■ Fill-in-the-Blank

1. The process of heating fermented mixtures of cereal grains or fruits in a still to evaporate and be trapped as purified alcohol is called ______________________________.

2. A drug that blocks sensitivity to pain is an ______________________________.

3. The principal enzyme that metabolizes ethanol is ______________________________

______________________________.

4. The concurrent use of multiple drugs is called ______________________________.

5. ______________________________ is the loss of conditioned reflexes due to depression of inhibitory centers of the brain.

6. A drug or substance that increases the production of urine is a ____________________.

7. ______________________________ is a psychotic condition connected with heavy alcohol use and associated vitamin deficiencies.

■ Identify

1. Identify four negative consequences of drinking alcohol.

a. ______________________________

b. ______________________________

c. ______________________________

d. ______________________________

2. Identify four negative consequences of drinking by college students.

a. ______________________________

b. ______________________________

c. ______________________________

d. ______________________________

3. Identify three possible explanations for why underage drinking increases the likelihood of developing dependence on alcohol.

a. ______________________________

b. ______________________________

c. ______________________________

4. Identify four factors that determine how alcohol will affect an individual's body.

a. ______________________________

b. ______________________________

c. ______________________________

d. ______________________________

5. Identify and describe the three prototypic stages of withdrawal.

a. ______________________________

b. ______________________________

c. ______________________________

6. Identify three medications that have been approved to treat alcoholism.

a. ______________________________

b. ______________________________

c. ______________________________

7. Describe three ways that genetics can increase the vulnerability to alcohol addiction.

a. ______________________________

b. ______________________________

c. ______________________________

8. Describe the three phases of alcohol-induced liver disease.

a. ______________________________

b. ______________________________

c. ______________________________

9. Describe how alcohol consumption affects each of the following:

a. Digestive system ______________________________

____

b. Blood ______________________________

____

c. Cardiovascular system ______________________________

____

d. Sexual organs ______________________________

____

e. Endocrine system ______________________________

____

f. Kidneys ______________________________

____

g. Brain ______________________________

____

h. Fetus ______________________________

____

____

■ Matching

Match the type of alcohol with its description.

_____ Methyl alcohol	a. Rubbing alcohol
_____ Ethylene glycol	b. Alcohol used in beverages
_____ Isopropyl alcohol	c. Wood alcohol
_____ Ethyl alcohol	d. Alcohol used as antifreeze

True/False

Tell whether each statement is true or false. If false, explain why the statement is incorrect.

1. Alcohol is a widely used and abused psychoactive drug. ______________________________

____

2. It is estimated that at some time during their lives, almost 50% of all Americans will be involved in an alcohol-related traffic accident. ______________________________

____

3. A recent study found that the consumption of 1.5 drinks accounts for 30% of the approximate 20,000 alcohol-linked cancers in the United States each year. ______________________________

____

4. Drinking black coffee or taking a cold shower will hasten the sobering process. ______________________________

____

5. Approximately 2000 college student deaths occur each year. ______________________________

____

6. Most alcohol use starts during the teen years. ______________________________

____

Discussion Questions

1. Why is alcohol perceived as acceptable for social use as well as for relieving stress and anxiety? Why do many people often forget alcohol's harmful consequences? ______________________________

____

____

____

____

2. What are some possible reasons why people use alcohol with other drugs, like marijuana? ______________________________

____

____

____

____

3. What is meant by "taking the hair of the dog that bit you"? Is this an effective method of reducing hangovers? Why or why not? ______

4. How can knowledge of the role of genetics in alcoholism help deal with the problem? ______

5. What does current scientific evidence say about the relationship between alcohol consumption and cancer? ______

Notes

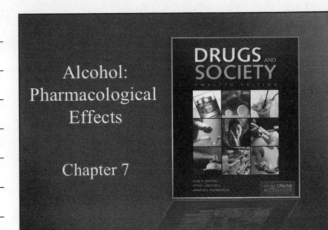

Alcohol as a Drug

- Alcohol is a psychoactive drug that is a CNS depressant.
- Some claim that alcohol is the most widely consumed drug in the world and for some is as much a part of daily life as eating.

Alcohol as a Drug (continued)

- Alcohol is an addictive substance. Of the approximately 2 million receiving treatment for drug abuse, 64% are being treated for alcoholism.
- Social psychologists refer to the perception of alcohol as a social lubricant.
- Four reasons why many people view alcohol as a non-drug:
  - Alcohol is legal.
  - Advertising and media promote drinking as normal.
  - Large distribution and sales of alcohol.
  - Long history of alcohol use.

Notes

Negative Impact of Alcohol

- 100,000 deaths associated with alcohol each year.
- Nearly 50% of all Americans will be involved in an alcohol-related traffic accident sometime during their lives.
- More than 2% of night-time drivers have blood alcohol that exceeds legal amounts (0.08%).

Negative Impact of Alcohol (continued)

- Alcohol causes severe dependence.
- Disrupts personal, family, social, and professional functioning.
- Illness, accidents, violence, and crime related to alcohol use.
- Consumption by college students causes approximately 2,000 deaths per year.

Negative Impact of Alcohol (continued)

- Fetal alcohol syndrome.
- Alcohol is the second leading cause of premature death in America.
- Approximately $250 billion is spent annually dealing with social and health problems related to alcohol use.

Four Types of Alcohol

- Methyl alcohol (poisonous)
- Isopropyl alcohol (poisonous)
- Ethylene glycol (poisonous)
- Ethanol (drinking alcohol)

Physical Effects of Alcohol

- The body is affected by alcohol in two ways:
  - Direct contact in mouth, esophagus, stomach, and intestine
  - Influence on almost every organ system in the body after entering the bloodstream
- Absorption is the process by which the drug molecules reach the bloodstream.
- The effects of alcohol on the human body depend on the blood alcohol content (BAC).

Physical Effects of Alcohol (continued)

- BAC produced depends on
  - Presence of food in the stomach
  - Rate of alcohol consumption
  - Concentration of alcohol
  - Drinker's body composition
- Alcoholic beverages have no vitamins, minerals, protein, or fat—just a large amount of carbohydrates and associated calories.

Notes

Notes

Physical Effects of Alcohol (continued)

- Alcohol can cause severe physical and psychological dependence.
  - **Cross-tolerance**
  - **Behavioral tolerance:** Compensation of motor impairments through behavioral pattern modification by chronic alcohol users

Blood Alcohol Concentration (BAC)

- Almost 95% of consumed alcohol is inactivated by liver metabolism.
- The liver metabolizes alcohol at a slow and constant rate and is unaffected by the amount ingested.
- Thus, if one can of beer is consumed each hour, the BAC will remain constant.

How Alcohol Is Absorbed in the Body

1. **Mouth**—Alcohol is consumed orally.
2. **Stomach**—Alcohol goes right into the stomach. A little of the alcohol passes through the wall of the stomach and into the bloodstream. Most of the alcohol continues down into the small intestine.
3. **Small intestine**—Alcohol goes from the stomach into the small intestine. Most of the alcohol is absorbed through the walls of the intestine and into the bloodstream.
4. **Bloodstream**—The bloodstream carries the alcohol to all parts of the body, such as the brain, heart, and liver.
5. **Liver**—As the bloodstream carries the alcohol around the body, it passes through the liver. The liver changes the alcohol to water, carbon dioxide, and energy. The process is called oxidation. The liver can oxidize only about one-half ounce of alcohol per hour. Thus, until the liver has time to oxidize all of the alcohol, the alcohol continues passing through all parts of the body, including the brain.
6. **Brain**—Alcohol goes to the brain almost as soon as it is consumed. It continues passing through the brain until the liver oxidizes all the alcohol into carbon dioxide, water, and energy.

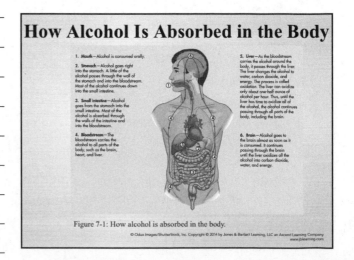

Figure 7-1: How alcohol is absorbed in the body.

Polydrug Use

- The common practice of taking alcohol concurrently with other drugs.

Polydrug Use (continued)

- Reasons why individuals may combine alcohol with other drugs:
  - Alcohol enhances properties of other CNS depressants.
  - Decreases the amount of an expensive and difficult-to-get drug required to achieve the desired effect.
  - Helps diminishes side effects of other drugs.
  - There is a common predisposition to use alcohol and other drugs.

Short-Term Effects of Alcohol

- Low to moderate doses
  - Disinhibition
  - Social setting and mental state may determine individual response
    - Euphoric, friendly, and talkative
    - Aggressive and hostile
  - Interfere with motor activity, reflexes, and coordination

Notes

Notes

Short-Term Effects of Alcohol (continued)

- Moderate quantities
  - Slightly increases heart rate
  - Slightly dilates blood vessels in arms, legs, and skin
  - Moderately lowers blood pressure
  - Stimulates appetite
  - Increases production of gastric secretions
  - Increases urine output

Short-Term Effects of Alcohol (continued)

- At higher doses
  - Social setting has little influence on effects
  - Difficulty in walking, talking, and thinking
  - Induces drowsiness and causes sleep
  - Induces a hangover when drinking stops

Short-Term Effects of Alcohol (continued)

- Large amounts consumed rapidly
  - Severe depression of the brain system and motor control area of the brain
    - Lack of coordination, confusion, and disorientation
    - Stupor, anesthesia, coma, or death
- Lethal level of alcohol between 0.4 and 0.6 by volume in the blood

True or False?

- Drinking black coffee, taking a cold shower, or breathing pure oxygen will hasten the sobering up process.
- The type of alcohol beverage you drink can influence the hangover that results.
- Taking an aspirin-caffeine combination after drinking helps the sobering up process and the chances of having a hangover.

Principle Control Centers of the Brain Affected by Alcohol

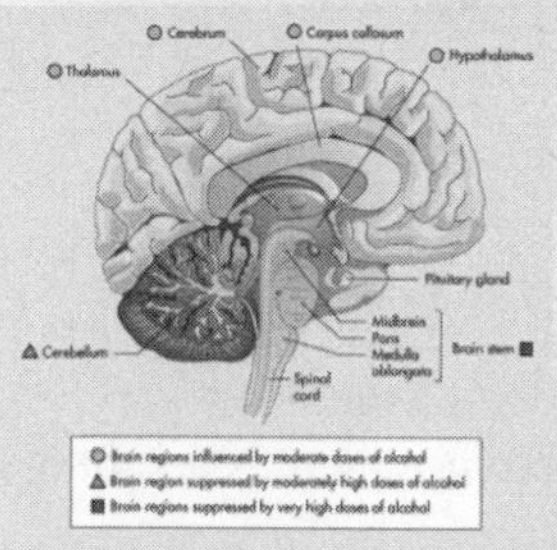

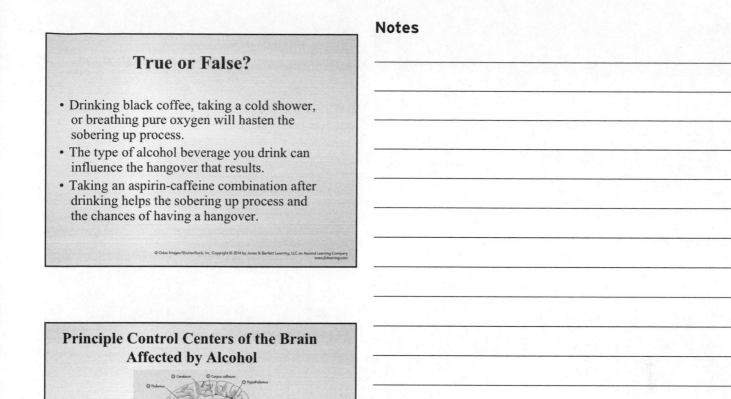

Figure 7-2: The principal control centers of the brain affected by alcohol consumption. Note that all areas of the brain are interconnected.

Dependence

- 12.5 million alcoholics in United States
- Approximately 50% high school seniors get drunk annually
- Recovered alcoholics are more likely to relapse when under stress
- Recovery from alcoholism is a long-term process

Notes

Notes

Medications for Alcohol Dependence

• Disulfiram (Antabuse): Makes alcohol very unpleasant by altering its metabolism
• Natrexone (opiate antagonist): Helps relieve craving in 20% of alcoholics
• Acamprosate (Campral): Reduces withdrawal in abstinent alcoholics

Alcohol and Genetics

- Alcoholism is among the most inherited mental illnesses
- Specific genes contribute to: (i) excessive consumption, (ii) diminished negative feedback, (iii) enhanced sense of pleasure, and (iv) diminished hangovers
- However, environment is as important as genetics

Effects of Alcohol on Organ Systems and Bodily Functions

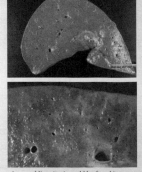

• Brain and nervous system
• Liver
  - Hepatotoxic effect
  - Alcoholic hepatitis
  - Cirrhosis
• Digestive system

A normal liver (top) would be found in a healthy human body. An abnormal liver (bottom) that exhibits the effects of moderate to heavy alcohol consumption.

Courtesy of CDC/ Dr. Edwin P. Ewing, Jr.

Effects of Alcohol on Organ Systems and Bodily Functions (continued)

- Blood
- Cardiovascular system
  - Alcoholic cardiomyopathy
- Sexual organs
- Endocrine system

Effects of Alcohol on Organ Systems and Bodily Functions (continued)

- Kidneys
- Mental disorder and damage to the brain
  - Wernicke-Korsakoff's syndrome
- The fetus
  - Fetal alcohol syndrome (FAS)

Alcohol and Pregnancy

- Moderate to excessive drinking during pregnancy can result in:
  - Spontaneous abortion
  - Damage to fetus
    - Fetal alcohol syndrome (FAS)
      - Damage dose-related
      - **A safe lower level of alcohol consumption has not been established for pregnant women**

Notes

Notes

Other Effects of Alcohol on Organ Systems and Bodily Functions

- Gender differences
- Malnutrition

CHAPTER 8

Alcohol: Behavioral Effects

The chapter outline provides you with an organizational guide to the topics and ideas presented in this chapter of the text.

Introduction
Alcohol Consumption in the United States
Current Statistics and Trends in Alcohol Consumption
- Percentages of the Drinking Population: A Pyramid Model
- Dual Problems: Underage and Adult Drinking
- Economic Costs of Alcohol Abuse

History of Alcohol in America
- Drinking Patterns
- Historical Considerations

Defining Alcoholics
- Cultural Differences
- Alcohol Abuse and Alcoholism
- Types of Alcoholics
- Major Traditional Distinctions Between "Wet" and "Dry" Cultures

Cultural Influences
- Culture and Drinking Behavior
- Culture and Disinhibited Behavior
- Culture Provides Rules for Drinking Behavior
- Culture Provides Ceremonial Meaning for Alcohol Use
- Culture Provides Models of Alcoholism
- Cultural Stereotypes of Drinking May Be Misleading
- Culture Provides Attitudes Regarding Alcohol Consumption

College and University Students and Alcohol Use
- Binge Drinking
- Gender and Collegiate Alcohol Use

Alcohol Consumption Patterns of Women
- The Role of Alcohol in Domestic Violence
- Alcohol and Sex

Alcohol and the Family: Destructive Types of Social Support and Organizations for Victims of Alcoholics
- Codependency and Enabling
- Children of Alcoholics and Adult Children of Alcoholics

Treatment of Alcoholism
- Getting Through Withdrawal
- Helping the Alcoholic Family Recover

Key Terms

Define the following terms:

1. **Binge use (binge drinking)** ______________________________
2. **Heavy use** ______________________________
3. **Teetotalers** ______________________________
4. **Bootlegging** ______________________________
5. **Drunken comportment** ______________________________
6. **Pseudointoxicated** ______________________________
7. **Relapsing syndrome** ______________________________
8. **Acute alcohol withdrawal syndrome** ______________________________

   ____
9. **Delirium tremens** ______________________________
10. **Psychodrama** ______________________________
11. **Post-traumatic stress disorder** ______________________________

    ____

Fill-in-the-Blank

1. Men who drink five or more alcoholic beverages and women who drink four or more drinks on one occasion are ______________________________.
2. Places where alcoholic beverages were illegally sold during the Prohibition era were called ______________________________.
3. The ingredients in ______________________________ were secret, often consisting of large amounts of colored water, alcohol, cocaine, or opiates.
4. ______________________________ is uncontrollable drinking that leads to alcohol craving, loss of control, and physical dependence but with less prominent characteristics than found in ______________________________, which is a state of physical and psychological addiction to ethanol.
5. A ______________________________ is a psychoactive chemical that depresses thought and judgment functions in the cerebral cortex, which has the effect of allowing relatively unrestrained behavior.
6. ______________________________ refers to the individual's expectation of what a drug will do to his or her personality; ______________________________ is the physical and social environments where the drug is consumed.

7. Unplanned and unwanted forced sexual attack from a friend or date partner is known as ______________________________.

8. ______________________ is a therapeutic technique in which group members play assigned parts to elicit emotional reactions.

9. A family therapy technique that records information about behavior and relationships on a type of family tree to elucidate persistent patterns of dysfunctional behavior is a ______________________.

■ Identify

1. Identify three major developments that occurred as a result of Prohibition.
   a. ______________________
   b. ______________________
   c. ______________________

2. Identify and define four major components of alcoholism.
   a. ______________________
   b. ______________________
   c. ______________________
   d. ______________________

3. Identify and describe Jellinek's six categories of alcoholism.
   a. ______________________
   b. ______________________
   c. ______________________
   d. ______________________
   e. ______________________
   f. ______________________

4. Identify three reasons why women respond differently than men to alcohol.

a. ______________________________

b. ______________________________

c. ______________________________

5. Identify two ways family members give destructive support to alcohol addicts. Explain and give an example of each.

a. ______________________________

____

b. ______________________________

____

6. Identify three ways in which the treatment of alcoholism differs from the treatment of other drug addictions.

a. ______________________________

b. ______________________________

c. ______________________________

■ Discussion Questions

1. A large percentage of those who drink alcohol are below the legal drinking age of 21. Do you think the drinking age should be lowered? Why or why not? ______________________________

____

____

____

2. What is the cost of alcohol abuse on society? Give multiple examples. ______________________________

____

____

____

3. How did the slave trade contribute to colonial America's alcohol production? ______________________________

____

____

____

4. Why is it difficult to establish one universal definition of alcoholism?

5. How does one's culture influence behavior regarding the use and abuse of alcohol?

6. How do cultures other than America view drinking? Discuss a different culture and the ways in which that culture approaches alcohol.

7. Why are alcohol use and binge drinking so prevalent on college campuses?

8. In what ways does alcoholism affect one's entire family? How does the family react and adapt to having an alcoholic member? What help is available to the family of an alcoholic?

Notes

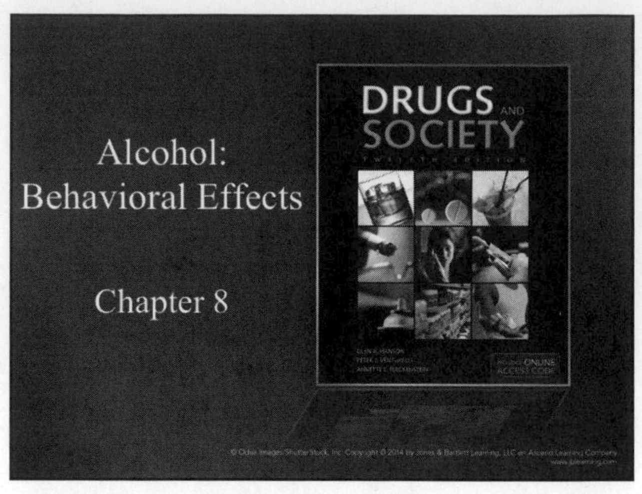
Alcohol:
Behavioral Effects
Chapter 8
DRUGS AND SOCIETY

How Serious Is Alcohol Consumption?

- Approximately 51.8% (133.4 million) of Americans are past-month alcohol drinkers (also referred to as current drinkers).
- Approximately 22.6% (58.3 million) of Americans binge drink and 6.2% (15.9 million) reported heavy drinking.

How Serious is Alcohol Consumption? (continued)

- Alcohol use (age 12 or older):
  - 56.8% of whites
  - 46.9% of persons reporting two or more races
  - 44.7% of American Indians or Alaska Natives
  - 42.5% of Hispanics
  - 42.1% of blacks
  - 40% of Asians

How Serious Is Alcohol Consumption? (continued)

- Estimated spending for yearly healthcare services for alcohol problems and medical consequences of alcohol: $18.8 billion.
- Alcohol is officially linked to at least half of all highway fatalities.
- To date, alcohol has been tried by 38.9% of 8th graders, 58.3% of 10th graders, 78.9% of 12th graders, and 83.5% of college students.
- An estimated yearly $82 billion was lost in potential productivity due to alcohol and other drug use.

How Serious is Alcohol Consumption?

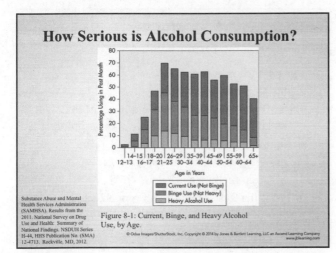

Substance Abuse and Mental Health Services Administration (SAMHSA). Results from the 2011. National Survey on Drug Use and Health: Summary of National Findings. NSDUH Series H-44, HHS Publication No. (SMA) 12-4713. Rockville, MD, 2012.

Figure 8-1: Current, Binge, and Heavy Alcohol Use, by Age.

Alcohol and Marijuana Use and the Very Young

- Use of alcohol to the point of inebriation: 18% of 8th graders, 37% of 10th graders, and 55% of 12 graders.
- Self-reported drunkenness 30 days prior to being surveyed: 5% of 8th, 14%, of 10th, and 30% of 12th graders.
- On a daily basis for 8th, 10th, and 12th graders, marijuana usage now exceeds alcohol usage.
- 42.6% of all 12th graders reported some marijuana use in their lifetime (34% reported past year and 20% reported past month).

Notes

Notes

History of Alcohol (Ethanol) in America

- 1830: Peak drinking period
- Prohibition period
- Alcohol has coincided with historical events:
  - Colonial America
  - Triangle trade (New England Yankees traded rum for slaves in Africa, then slaves for molasses in West Indies, and then back to New England to make rum)
  - Colonial taverns were key "institutions" promoting alcohol consumption

History of Alcohol in America (continued)

- Temperance movement (1830–1850)
- Prohibition era (1920–1933)
  - Ratification of the 18th Amendment (1919) to the U.S. Constitution (outlawing alcohol use)
  - Alcohol was outlawed (January 1920)
    - Speakeasies and bootlegging grew
    - Patent medicines flourished
- In 1933, the 21st Amendment repealed Prohibition

Major Problems Encountered During Prohibition Period

1. Alcohol use began to diminish for the first 2 or 3 years after Prohibition was in effect. However, after 3 years of steady decline, the use of distilled liquors rose every year afterward.
2. Enforcement against alcohol use was overthrown by corruption in law enforcement.
3. Many early European immigrants populating American cities during Prohibition came from cultures that viewed drinking as normal and customary, resulting in their refusal to give up alcohol consumption.

Defining Alcoholism

- There is no agreement regarding at what specific point someone is an alcoholic.
- Alcoholism is a state of physical and psychological addiction to a psychoactive substance known as ethanol.
- Most definitions include chronic behavioral disorders, repeated drinking to the point of loss of control, health disorders, and difficulty functioning socially and economically.

Defining Alcoholism: First Definition

World Health Organization (WHO) definition:

- "*Alcohol dependence syndrome* is characterized by a state, psychic and usually also physical, resulting from drinking alcohol. This state is characterized by behavioral and other responses that include a compulsion to take alcohol on a continuous or periodic basis to experience its psychic effects and sometimes to avoid the discomfort of its absence; tolerance may or may not be present" (NIAAA, 1980).

Defining Alcoholism: Second Definition

- "Alcoholism is a chronic behavioral disorder manifested by repeated drinking of alcoholic beverages in excess of the dietary and social uses of the community, and to an extent that interferes with the drinker's health or his social or economic functioning" (Keller, 1958).

Notes

Notes

Defining Alcoholism: Third Definition

- "Alcoholism is a chronic, primary, hereditary disease that progresses from an early, physiological susceptibility into an addiction characterized by tolerance changes, physiological dependence, and loss of control over drinking. Psychological symptoms are secondary to the physiological disease and not relevant to its onset''
(Gold, 1991).

Major Known Components of Alcoholism

- **Craving:** A compulsion to drink alcohol even during inappropriate times (e.g., while driving, working, at a formal event)
- **Very impaired or loss of control:** Inability to limit drinking once begun
- **Physical dependence:** Withdrawal symptoms when attempting to abstain (e.g., nausea, sweating, anxiety)
- **Tolerance:** Need to increase usage to achieve the effect, the "buzz" from alcohol

Types of Alcoholics by Jellinek

- **Alpha alcoholics:** Mostly a psychological dependence
- **Beta alcoholics:** Mostly socially dependent on alcohol
- **Gamma alcoholics:** Most severe; suffers from emotional and psychological impairment
- **Delta alcoholics:** Constantly losing control over the amount of alcohol consumed
- **Epsilon alcoholics:** Constantly binge drinking and at times days at a time
- **Zeta alcoholics:** Moderate drinker who becomes abusive and violent

Types of Alcoholics by Moss et al.

- **Young Adult** (31.5% of U.S. alcoholics): Young adult drinkers without major problems regarding their drinking
- **Young Antisocial** (21% of U.S. alcoholics): Mid-20s, had earlier onset of regular drinking and alcohol problems, and come from heavy alcohol use families
- **Functional** (19.5% of U.S. alcoholics): Middle-aged, well-educated, with stable jobs and families
- **Intermediate Familial** (19% of U.S. alcoholics): Middle-aged, with 50% from families with multigenerational alcoholism
- **Chronic Severe** (9% of U.S. alcoholics): Mostly middle-aged, high rates of antisocial personality disorder and criminality

Culture and Alcohol: Important Terms

- **Drunken comportment:** Behavior exhibited while under the direct influence of alcohol determined by the norms and expectations of a particular culture.
- **Disinhibitor:** A psychoactive chemical that depresses thought and judgment functions in the cerebral cortex, which has the effect of allowing relatively unrestrained behavior (as in alcohol inebriation).
- **Pseudointoxication:** Acting inebriated even before the quantity consumed produces its effects.

Culture and Alcohol (continued)

- Some psychologists contend that both *set and setting* can often overshadow the pharmacological effects of most drugs, including alcohol.
  - **Set:** An individual's expectation of what a drug will do to his/her personality
  - **Setting:** The physical and social environment where most drugs, including alcohol, are consumed

Notes

Notes

Culture and Alcohol

- Culture provides how alcohol use is perceived (e.g., violation of norms, "normal" to drink, sexy, sophisticated, mature).
- Cultural rules state how much one can drink and where one can drink.
- Cultures provide ceremonial meaning to alcohol use.
  - Drinking rates among Jews
  - Drinking rates among Irish
- Culture provides a model of alcoholism.
- Culture provides attitudes and stereo-types regarding drinking behavior.

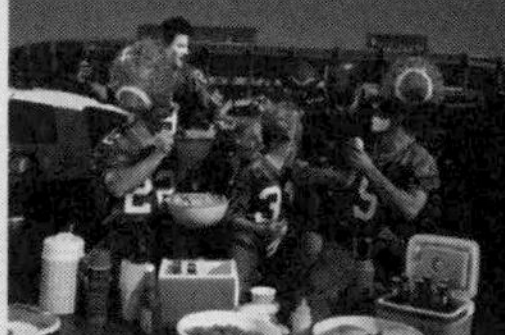

Alcohol consumption is routine at many social activities for college students.

© Nice One Productions/age fotostock

Distinctions Between "Wet" and "Dry Cultures

- **"Wet" Cultures** - In these cultures alcohol is integrated into daily life and activities (e.g., alcohol consumed with meals). In these cultures, abstinence rates are low and wine is largely the beverage of preference. European countries bordering the Mediterranean have traditionally exemplified wet cultures.
- **"Dry" Cultures** – Alcohol consumption is not as common during everyday activities. Abstinence is more common, however, when drinking occurs, it is more likely to result in intoxication. Scandinavian countries, the U.S., and Canada are examples of counties that are dry.

Alcohol Abuse Among College and University Students

CORE Institute (2008) research results:

- Approximately 72% of college students consumed alcohol and 42% to 55% engaged in binge drinking within 30 days when survey was given.
- College students consume an average of 5.4 alcoholic drinks per week.
- Of all the drugs reported, alcohol was the most heavily abused on college campuses, followed by tobacco (44%) and marijuana (31%).

Notes

Alcohol Abuse Among College and University Students (continued)

Other studies found that ...

- The main reason given for binge drinking was "to get drunk."
- Males binge drink more than females.
- For binge drinkers, the impact on impaired academic performance is just as great for women drinkers.
- Being white, involved in athletics, or a resident of a fraternity or sorority made it more likely that a student would be a binge drinker.

Alcohol Abuse Among College and University Students

- On U.S. campuses, alcohol is a factor in 40% of all academic problems and 28% of all dropouts.
- Seventy-five percent of male students and 55% of female students involved in acquaintance rape had been drinking or using drugs.
- The transition into college is associated with a doubling of the percentages of those who drink for both males and females.
- For heavier drinkers, grades suffered for both male and female students.

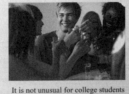

It is not unusual for college students overconsume alcohol when they are partying.

Women and Alcohol

- Women possess greater sensitivity to alcohol, have a greater likelihood of addiction, and develop alcohol-related health problems sooner than men (e.g., stomach cancer, cirrhosis of the liver).
- More women in alcohol treatment come from sexually abusive homes (70%) in comparison to men (12%).

Notes

Women and Alcohol (continued)

- Three major reasons why women are more sensitive to the effects of alcohol:
  1. Body size (men generally larger than women)
  2. Women absorb alcohol sooner—women possess more body fat and body fat does not dilute alcohol
  3. Women possess less of a metabolizing enzyme that gets rid of (processes out) alcohol

Women and Alcohol (continued)

- Alcohol consumption patterns of women:
  - Women 21 to 34 years of age were least likely to report alcohol-related problems if they had stable marriages and were working full time.
  - Women tend to marry men whose drinking habits match their own.
  - Between 35 to 49 years of age, the heaviest drinkers were divorced or separated women without children.
  - Between 50 to 64 years of age, the heaviest drinkers were women whose husbands/partners drank heavily.
  - Women 65 and older comprised less than 10% of drinkers with drinking problems.

Alcohol Consumption in the United States

- Alcohol consumption has dropped sharply since 1981.
- What explains the steady decline in alcohol consumption during the past twenty years?
  - Demographics
  - Conservatism
  - Decrease in social acceptability
  - Increased awareness of risks
  - Increased concerns for health

Additional Facts Regarding Alcohol Use/Abuse

- Drinking and driving: On most weekend nights throughout the United States, 70% of all fatal single-vehicle crashes involve a driver who is legally intoxicated.
- Income/wealth: Less affluent people drink less than more affluent individuals.
- The average "alcoholic": The largest percentage of alcoholics are secret or disguised drinkers who look very much like common working people.
- On average: Most people who consume alcohol do not become problem drinkers.

Alcohol and the Family

- **Co-dependency** (or *co-alcoholism*): A relationship pattern in which addicted or nonaddicted family members identify with the alcohol addict and deny the existence of alcohol consumption as a problem.
- **Enabling:** Denial or making up of excuses for the excessive drinking of an alcohol addict to whom someone is close.

Alcohol and the Family (continued)

- Children of alcoholics (COAs) 2–4 times more likely to become alcoholics themselves.
- Adult children of alcoholics (ACOAs) 2–4 times more likely to develop alcoholism.
- Approximately, 9.7 million children age 17 or younger are living in households with one or more adults classified as having an alcohol abuse or dependence problem.
  - Seventy percent of these children were biological, foster, adopted, or stepchildren.
  - As a result, 6.8 million children, or about 15% of children aged 17 or younger, meet the formal definition of children of alcoholics.
- COAs and ACOAs are more likely to marry into families where alcoholism is prevalent.
- Twenty-five percent of American children are exposed to an alcoholic before the age of 18.

Notes

Notes

Helping the Family Recover

- **Psychodrama:** A family therapy in which significant inter- and intra-personal issues are enacted in a focused setting using dramatic techniques.
- **Genogram:** A family therapy technique that records information about behavior and relationships on a type of family tree to elucidate persistent patterns of dysfunctional behavior.
- **Role-playing:** A therapeutic technique in which group members play assigned parts to elicit emotional actors.

Helping the Family Recover
(continued)

- **Post-traumatic stress disorder:** A psychiatric syndrome in which an individual who has been exposed to a traumatic event or situation experiences psychological stress that may manifest itself in a wide range of symptoms, including re-experiencing the trauma, numbing of general responsiveness, and hyper-arousal.

Recovery from Alcoholism

- Treatment of alcoholism
  - Denial as a psychological defense
  - Easy to relapse without radical shift in lifestyle
  - Alcohol rehabilitation and medical ramifications
  - More emotionally fragile than other addicts
  - *Relapsing syndrome*

Withdrawal
• **Relapsing syndrome:** Returning to the use of alcohol after quitting.
• **Acute alcohol withdrawal syndrome:** Symptoms that occur when an alcohol addicted individual does not maintain his/her usual blood alcohol level.
• **Delirium tremens:** The most severe, even life-threatening, form of alcohol withdrawal, involving hallucinations, deliriums, and fever.

Notes

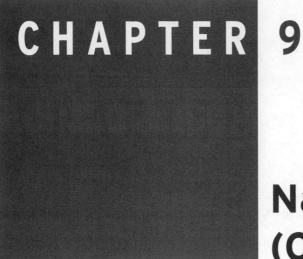

CHAPTER 9

Narcotics (Opioids)

The chapter outline provides you with an organizational guide to the topics and ideas presented in this chapter of the text.

Introduction
What Are Narcotics?
The History of Narcotics
- Opium in China
- American Opium Use

Pharmacological Effects
- Narcotic Analgesics
- Other Therapeutic Uses
- Abuse of Prescription Opioid Painkillers
- Mechanisms of Action
- Side Effects

Abuse, Tolerance, Dependence, and Withdrawal
- Heroin Abuse
- Patterns of Heroin Abuse
- Treatment of Heroin and Other Narcotic Dependence

Other Narcotics
- Morphine
- Methadone
- Fentanyls
- Hydromorphone
- Oxycodone
- Meperidine
- Buprenorphine
- MPTP: A "Designer" Tragedy
- Codeine
- Pentazocine
- Propoxyphene
- Tramadol

Narcotic-Related Drugs
- Dextromethorphan
- Clonidine
- Naloxone/Naltrexone

Natural Narcotic Substances

Key Terms

Define the following terms:

1. **Analgesics** ____________________
2. **Opioid** ____________________
3. **Antitussive** ____________________
4. **Speedballing** ____________________

Fill-in-the-Blank

1. ______________________ are drugs that are derived from opium.
2. Drugs that block coughing are ______________________.
3. To ______________________ is to inject a drug of abuse intravenously.
4. ______________________ are the most likely type of prescription drugs to be abused.

Identify

1. Identify three therapeutic uses for narcotics.
   a. ______________________
   b. ______________________
   c. ______________________
2. What are some possible side effects of opioid narcotics? ______________________
   ____
   ____
   ____
3. Identify and describe the two major stages in the development of a psychological dependence on heroin or other opioid narcotics.
   a. ______________________
   b. ______________________
4. Identify six goals of heroin dependency treatment.
   a. ______________________
   b. ______________________
   c. ______________________
   d. ______________________
   e. ______________________
   f. ______________________
5. What are the three medications approved by the FDA for the treatment of heroin addictions?
   a. ______________________
   b. ______________________
   c. ______________________

■ Matching

Match the drug with its description.

____ Morphine

____ Methadone

____ Fentanyls

____ Meperidine

____ Buprenorphine

____ Tramadol

____ Codeine

____ Pentazocine

____ Propoxyphene

____ Dextromethorphan

____ Clonidine

____ Naloxone/Naltrexone

____ Oxycodone

a. prepared from morphine and used as an analgesic and cough suppressant.

b. stimlulates receptors for noradrenaline; used to relieve some physical effects of opiate withdrawal; nonaddictive.

c. effective in relieving the cravings for narcotic pain relievers with diminished tendency to cause addiction itself.

d. often substituted for heroin in the treatment of severely narcotic-dependent people.

e. used by primary care physicians to treat opioid dependence in their own offices.

f. the active opioid ingredient in OxyContin.

g. synthetic used in cough remedies; no analgesic action.

h. an opioid analgesic with low risk of dependence; not scheduled by the FDA.

i. will precipitate withdrawal symptoms if given to a person on methadone maintenance; not commonly abused because its effects can be unpleasant, resulting in dysphoria.

j. relatively pure narcotic antagonists; prevent narcotic drugs from having an effect.

k. very weak analgesic; in very high doses, it can cause delusions, hallucinations, and convulsions.

l. very potent narcotic analgesics that are often administered intravenously for general anesthesia.

m. naturally occurring constituent of opium; prescribed as a potent narcotic analgesic.

n. synthetic drug frequently used for treatment of moderate pain; repeated high doses can cause seizures.

■ Discussion Questions

1. Discuss ways to treat heroin dependency. What are mistakes some people make when trying to treat this?

____

____

____

2. Why does heroin addiction often contribute to criminal activity? ________________

____

____

____

3. What are the benefits of using buprenorphine to treat opioid addiction? ________________

____

____

____

Notes

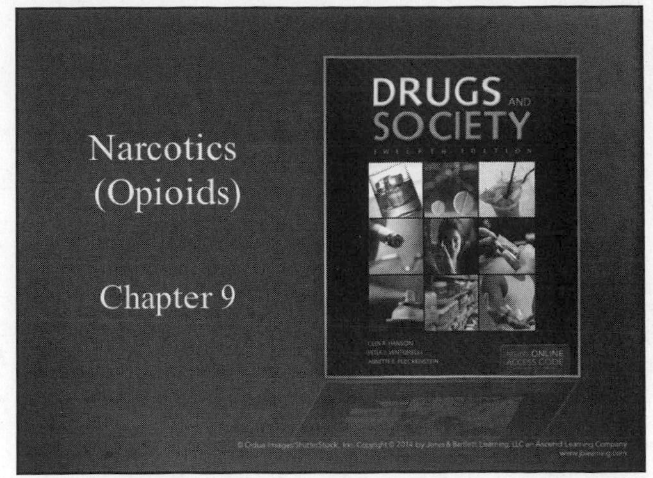

What Are Narcotics?

- The term *narcotic* currently refers to naturally occurring substances derived from the opium poppy and their synthetic substitutes.
- These drugs are referred to as the opioid (or opiate) narcotics because of their association with opium.

What Are Narcotics? (continued)

- Abuse rate for prescribed opioid narcotics has gone from 2.2% to 10% in the past 10 years
- Although opioid narcotics possess abuse potential, they also have important clinical value (e.g., analgesic, antitussive, antidiarrheal).
- The term *narcotic* has been used to label many substances, from opium to marijuana to cocaine.

Notes

The History of Narcotics

- A 6000-year-old Sumerian tablet
- The Egyptians
- The Greeks
- Arab traders
- China and opium trade
- The Opium War of 1839
- American opium use
- Abuse problems often associated with war

Pharmacological Effects

- The most common clinical use of the opioid narcotics is as analgesics to relieve pain.
- The opioid narcotics relieve pain by activating the same group of receptors that are controlled by the endogenous substances called *endorphins*.
- Activation of opioid receptors blocks the transmission of pain through the spinal cord or brain stem but can also reduce the effects of stress.

Pharmacological Effects (continued)

- *Morphine* is a particularly potent pain reliever and often is used as the analgesic standard by which other narcotics are compared.
- With continual use, tolerance develops to the analgesic effects of morphine and other narcotics.
- Physicians frequently underprescribe narcotics, for fear of causing narcotic addiction.

Pharmacological Effects (continued)

- The principle side effects of opioid narcotics, besides their abuse potential, include:
  - Drowsiness, mental clouding
  - Respiratory depression
  - Nausea, vomiting, and constipation
  - Inability to urinate
  - Drop in blood pressure

Abuse, Tolerance, Dependence, and Withdrawal

- All the opioid narcotic agents that activate opioid receptors have abuse potential and are classified as scheduled drugs.
- Tolerance begins with the first dose of a narcotic, but does not become clinically evident until after 2 to 3 weeks of frequent use.

Abuse of Opioid Narcotics

- Tolerance occurs most rapidly with high doses given in short intervals.
- Doses can be increased as much as 35 times in order to regain the narcotic effect.
- Physical dependence invariably accompanies severe tolerance and typically expresses when these drugs are used for more than 2–4 weeks.
- Psychological dependence can also develop with continual narcotic use.

Notes

Notes

Guidelines to Avoid Prescribed Opiate Abuse

- Only use opioid analgesics when pain severity warrants
- Doses and duration of use should be as conservative as possible
- Patients should store these medications securely to prevent their theft and misuse
- Do not share with anyone else
- Doctors should screen patients for abuse risk before prescribing opioid drugs

Guidelines to Avoid Prescribed Opiate Abuse (continued)

- Patients should be educated about potential abuse problems prior to being prescribed opioid drugs
- If significant abuse is suspected, the clinician should discuss concerns with patient to find appropriate steps to stop the abuse

Opioid Side Effects

- Drowsiness
- Respiratory depression
- Nausea/vomiting
- Inability to urinate
- Constricted pupils
- Constipation
- Physical dependence and withdrawal

Heroin Abuse

- Heroin is classified as a Schedule I drug.
  - One of the most widely abused illegal drugs in the world; accounts for >$120 billion sales/year
  - Illicitly used more than any other drug of abuse in the United States (except for marijuana) until 20 years ago, when it was replaced by cocaine
  - Some of the recent increases in heroin use likely due to increased abuse of prescription opioid painkillers

Heroin Combinations

- Pure heroin is a white powder.
- More than 90% of world's heroin is from Afghanistan.
- Heroin is usually "cut" (diluted) with **lactose**.
- When heroin first enters the United States, it may be 95% pure; by the time it is sold, it may be 3% to 70% pure.
- If users are unaware of the variance in purity and do not adjust doses accordingly, results can be fatal.

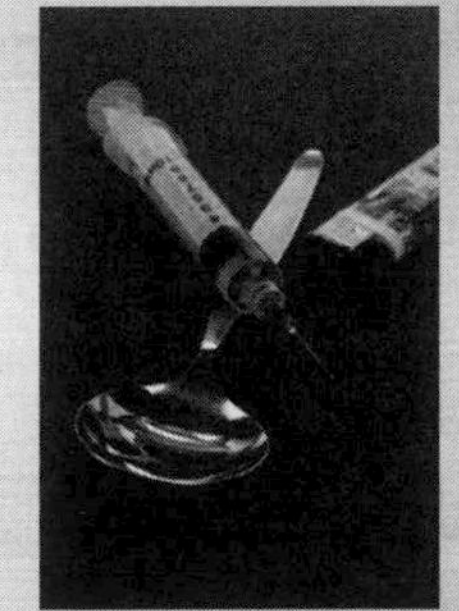

Heroin paraphernalia is usually simple and crude but effective: a spoon on which to dissolve the narcotic and a makeshift syringe with which to inject it.

Heroin Combinations (continued)

- Heroin has a bitter taste and is often cut with **quinine**, which can be a deadly adulterant.
- Heroin plus the artificial narcotic **fentanyl** can be dangerous due to its unexpected potency.
- Heroin is most frequently used with **alcohol**.
- Heroin combined with **cocaine** is called "speedballing."

Notes

Notes

Facts About Heroin Abuse

- What is the estimated number of heroin addicts in the United States?
  - 600,000
- What are "shooting galleries"?
  - Locations that serve as gathering places for addicts

Heroin and Crime

- Factors related to crime:
  - Pharmacological effects encourage antisocial behavior that is crime-related
  - Heroin diminishes inhibition
  - Addicts are often self-centered, impulsive, and governed by need
  - Cost of addiction
  - Similar personality of criminal and addict

Patterns of Heroin Abuse

- Heroin has become purer (60% to 70% purity) and cheaper (~$10/bag).
- Greater purity leads users to administer heroin in less efficient ways.
- Many youth believe that heroin can be used safely if not injected.

Patterns of Heroin Abuse (continued)

- Because of its association with popular fashions and entertainment, heroin has been viewed as glamorous and chic, especially by many young people, although lately this attitude has been changing.
- Emergency room visits due to narcotic overdoses were over 190,000 in 2009.

Stages of Dependence

- Initially, the effects of heroin are often unpleasant.
- Euphoria gradually overcomes the aversive effects.
- The positive feelings increase with narcotic use, leading to psychological dependence.
- In addition to psychological dependence, physical dependence occurs with daily use over a 2-week period.
- If the user abruptly stops taking the drug after physical dependence has developed, severe withdrawal symptoms result.

Methods of Administration

- Sniffing the powder
- Injecting it into a muscle (intramuscular)
- Smoking
- Mainlining (intravenous injection)

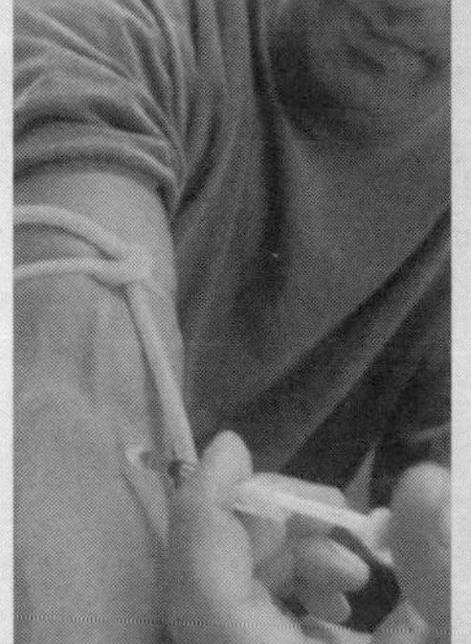

A heroin addict "mainlining" his drug.

Notes

Notes

Heroin Addicts and AIDS

- More than 250,000 patients in United States contracted AIDS by drug injection, of which most were heroin users.
- Fear of contracting HIV from IV heroin use has contributed to the increase in smoking or snorting heroin.
- Many who start by smoking or snorting progress to IV administration due to its more intense effects.

Heroin and Pregnancy

- Heroin use by a pregnant woman leads to:
  - Physical dependence on heroin in the newborn
  - Withdrawal symptoms after birth in the newborn (*Note:* similar withdrawal occurs in newborns of any woman who uses significant amounts of opiate drugs during pregnancy, including prescribed opiate painkillers)

Withdrawal Symptoms

- After the effects of the heroin wear off, the addicts have only a few hours in which to find the next dose before severe withdrawal symptoms begin.
- A single "shot" of heroin lasts 4 to 6 hours.
- Withdrawal symptoms: runny nose, tears, minor stomach cramps, loss of appetite, vomiting, diarrhea, abdominal cramps, chills, fever, aching bones, and muscle spasms.

Treatment

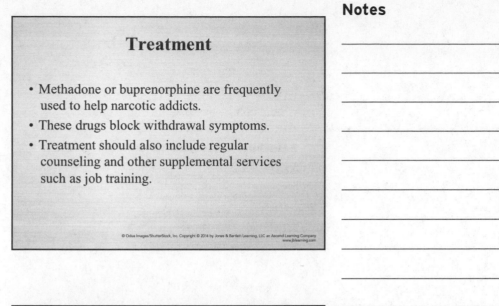

- Methadone or buprenorphine are frequently used to help narcotic addicts.
- These drugs block withdrawal symptoms.
- Treatment should also include regular counseling and other supplemental services such as job training.

Treatment

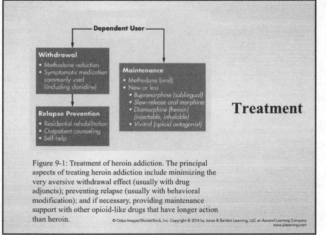

Figure 9-1: Treatment of heroin addiction. The principal aspects of treating heroin addiction include minimizing the very aversive withdrawal effect (usually with drug adjuncts); preventing relapse (usually with behavioral modification); and if necessary, providing maintenance support with other opioid-like drugs that have longer action than heroin.

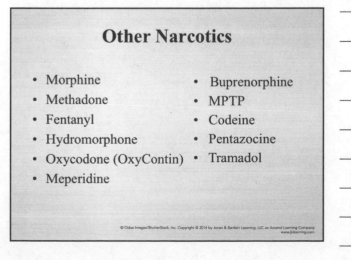

Other Narcotics

- Morphine
- Methadone
- Fentanyl
- Hydromorphone
- Oxycodone (OxyContin)
- Meperidine
- Buprenorphine
- MPTP
- Codeine
- Pentazocine
- Tramadol

Notes

Notes

Narcotic-Related Drugs

- **Dextromethorphan:** OTC antitussive
- **Clonidine:** Relieves some of the opioid withdrawal symptoms
- **Naloxone/Naltrexone:** Narcotic antagonist; used for narcotic overdoses

CHAPTER 10

Stimulants

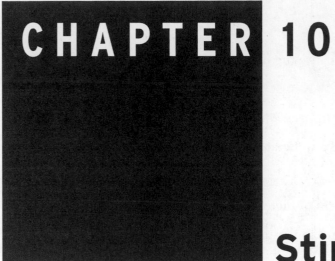

The chapter outline provides you with an organizational guide to the topics and ideas presented in this chapter of the text.

Introduction
Major Stimulants
- Amphetamines
- Cocaine

Minor Stimulants
- Caffeine-Like Drugs (Xanthines)
- OTC Sympathomimetics
- Herbal Stimulants

Global Stimulant Abuse
- Stimulant Production
- Stimulant Trafficking
- Global Stimulant Consumption
- Global Drug Policy

Key Terms

Define the following terms:

1. **Uppers** ______________________________
2. **Behavioral stereotypy** ______________________________
3. **Narcolepsy** ______________________________
4. **Speed** ______________________________
5. **Rush** ______________________________
6. **High** ______________________________
7. **Run** ______________________________
8. **Hyperpyrexia** ______________________________
9. **Freebasing** ______________________________
10. **Crack babies** ______________________________
11. **Xanthines** ______________________________
12. **Caffeinism** ______________________________

Fill-in-the-Blank

1. ______________________ are substances that cause the user to feel pleasant effects such as a sense of increased energy and a state of euphoria.
2. ______________________ are drugs that suppress one's appetite for food.
3. The two principal side effects of therapeutic doses of amphetamines are ______________________ and ______________________.
4. ______________________ is a smokable form of methamphetamine.
5. A ______________________ is similar to a run, but is usually of a shorter duration.
6. Repeated administration of methamphetamine to maintain the high is called ______________________.
7. Recruiting the help of many friends and associates to purchase legal amounts of the methamphetamine precursor chemicals such as pseudoephedrine (e.g., in decongestants) to sell to illegal methamphetamine producers is called ______________________.
8. Combinations of amphetamine or cocaine with an opioid narcotic are called ______________________.
9. Ecstasy is a ______________________, a drug used by young adults at dance parties such as raves.
10. When methylphenidate (Ritalin) is used by college students to increase physical or mental endurance to achieve a more positive outcome on exams, it is referred to as ______________________.
11. A drug is ______________________ when contaminating substances are mixed in to dilute the drug.
12. Already processed and inexpensive "freebased" cocaine, ready for smoking, is called ______________________.

Identify

1. Identify and briefly discuss the three approved uses of amphetamines.

   a. ______________________

   b. ______________________

   c. ______________________

2. Briefly discuss the three eras of cocaine history.

   a. The First Cocaine Era ______________________

   ____

b. The Second Cocaine Era ______________________________

____

c. The Third Cocaine Era______________________________

____

3. Describe the use and consequences of using methylphenidate by college students to help prepare for exams. ______________________________

____

____

4. Identify four street names for cocaine.

a. ______________________________

b. ______________________________

c. ______________________________

d. ______________________________

5. Identify four possible effects of cocaine withdrawal.

a. ______________________________

b. ______________________________

c. ______________________________

d. ______________________________

6. Give three reasons why the combined use of cocaine and alcohol can be so dangerous.

a. ______________________________

b. ______________________________

c. ______________________________

7. Explain why combining caffeine and alcohol in commercially prepared beverages is dangerous. ______

____

____

■ Discussion Questions

1. How were amphetamines put to use during wartime? Should they still be used today? ______________

____

____

____

2. How do amphetamines work in the body? ______________________________

3. What are some consequences of increased amphetamine use? ______________________________

4. How is amphetamine addiction treated? ______________________________

5. Why have local methamphetamine labs disappeared, and what has replaced them for supplying illegal methamphetamines? ______________________________

6. Why did the early South American civilizations have fewer negative experiences with cocaine use than we do now? ______________________________

7. How has American cocaine use affected South American countries? ______________________________

8. How can cocaine be administered? How does the method of use determine the intensity of the drug's effects? ______________________________

9. How is cocaine addiction treated? What are the major differences in treatment approaches? How does one determine which treatment is most appropriate for an addicted individual? ____________________

____

____

____

10. At what point does caffeine become dangerous? What effects does it have in higher doses? Should the FDA control it more tightly? ____________________

____

____

____

11. According to the World Health Organization, what does ATS stand for and how big of a global problem are they? ____________________

____

____

____

Notes

Stimulants

Chapter 10

DRUGS AND SOCIETY

Major Stimulants

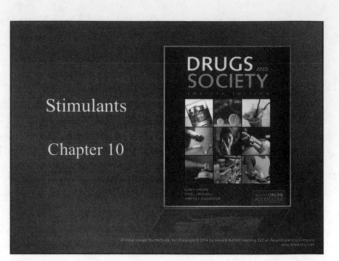

- All major stimulants increase alertness, excitation, and euphoria; thus, these drugs are referred to as "uppers."
  - Schedule I ("designer" amphetamines)
  - Schedule II (amphetamine, cocaine, methylphenicate-Ritalin)

Amphetamines

- Cause dependence due to their euphoric properties and ability to mask fatigue.
- Can be legally prescribed by physicians.
- Abuse occurs in people who acquire their drugs by both legitimate and illicit ways.

History of Amphetamines

- First synthesized in 1887 by L. Edeleano.
- In 1927, Gordon Alles gave a firsthand account of its effects.
  - Reduced fatigue
  - Increased alertness
  - Caused a sense of confident euphoria
- In 1932, Benzedrine inhalers became available as a nonprescription medication.

History of Amphetamines

- The Benzedrine inhalers became widely abused for their stimulant action.
  - 1971, all potent amphetamine-like compounds in nasal inhalers were withdrawn from the market.
- Widely used in World War II to counteract fatigue.
- Other users: Korean War soldiers, truck drivers, homemakers, high achievers under pressure (as performance-enhancers).

How Amphetamines Work

- Synthetic chemical similar to the natural neurotransmitters such as norepinephrine, dopamine, and epinephrine
- Increase the release and block the metabolism of these catecholamine substances, as well as serotonin, in the brain and peripheral nerves associated with the sympathetic nervous system

Notes

Notes

How Amphetamines Work (continued)

- Amphetamines can cause
  - "Fight-or-flight" effect, a response to crisis
  - Alertness
  - Anxiety, severe apprehension, or panic
  - Potent effects on dopamine in the reward center of the brain
  - **Behavioral stereotypy:** Meaningless repetition of a single activity

Approved Uses of Amphetamines

- Narcolepsy
- Attention Deficit Hyperactivity Disorder (ADHD)
- Weight reduction

Side Effects of Therapeutic Doses

- Abuse and addiction
- Cardiovascular toxicities
  - Increased heart rate
  - Elevated blood pressure
  - Damage to blood vessels

Current Misuse

- Decline in abuse in the late 1980s and early 1990s.
- In 1993 the declines were replaced by an increase.
- Currently, 3–6% annual use of methamphetamine by adolescents in the United States.
- Due to the ease of production, methamphetamine can be made in makeshift labs using cookbook-style recipes.
- Toxic chemicals in such labs pose a threat to residents, neighbors, law enforcement officials, and the environment.

Current Misuse (continued)

- Illegal labs that synthesize methamphetamine use decongestant ingredients from common OTC cold medicines.
- Role of the Comprehensive Methamphetamine Control Act 2008 in reducing illegal manufacturing of methamphetamine.
- Illicit neighborhood labs have been replaced by small local "shake and bake" and large Mexican drug cartel operations for methamphetamine supplies.

Patterns of High-Dose Use

- Amphetamines can be taken:
  - Orally
  - Intravenously (speed freak)
  - Smoked (ice)

Notes

Notes

Summary of the Effects of Amphetamines

	Body	Mind
low dose ↓ high dose	increased heartbeat, increased blood pressure, decreased appetite, increased breathing rate, inability to sleep, sweating, dry mouth, muscle twitching, convulsions, fever, chest pain, irregular heartbeat, death due to overdose	decreased fatigue, increased confidence, increased feeling of alertness, restlessness, talkativeness, increased irritability, fearfulness, apprehension, distrust of people, behavioral stereotypy, hallucination, psychosis

Amphetamines

- Amphetamine combinations
  - Speedballs
- Designer drugs
  - Methylenedioxymethamphetamine (MDMA, Ecstasy; most popular of the designer amphetamines)
  - Methylenedioxyamphetamine (MDA)
- A special amphetamine
  - Methylphenidate (Ritalin)

Treatment of Amphetamine Abuse

- Methamphetamine addiction is the principal problem with these drugs.
- Addiction causes long-term brain damage and is difficult, but not impossible, to treat.
- Requires long-term treatment to deal with compromised decision-making, memory deficits, increased impulsivity and lack of emotion control.
- No FDA-approved medications/treatment is principally behavioral management.

MDMA (Ecstasy)

- A designer amphetamine that continues to be popular with young people.
- It enhances sensory input and is referred to as an entactogen (a combination of psychedelic and stimulant effects) and it releases both serotonin and dopamine.
- While dependence can occur, it tends to be unusual.
- Withdrawal includes depression and sleep disruption that can last for days.

Performance Enhancers

- These are stimulants used to embellish physical/ mental endurance and enhance performance.
- Often used by college, and even high school, students to help academically.
- The drugs used can be illegal amphetamines or related prescription stimulants that are used to treat ADHD, like Ritalin.
- As with other potent stimulants, use of these drugs can be very dangerous and cause dependence.

Cocaine

- Cocaine abuse continues to be a major drug concern in the United States.
- From 1978 to 1987, the United States experienced the largest cocaine epidemic in history.
- As recently as the early 1980s cocaine was not believed to cause dependency.
- Cocaine is known to be highly addictive.
  - In 2010, approximately 2.4% of high school seniors used cocaine.

Notes

Notes

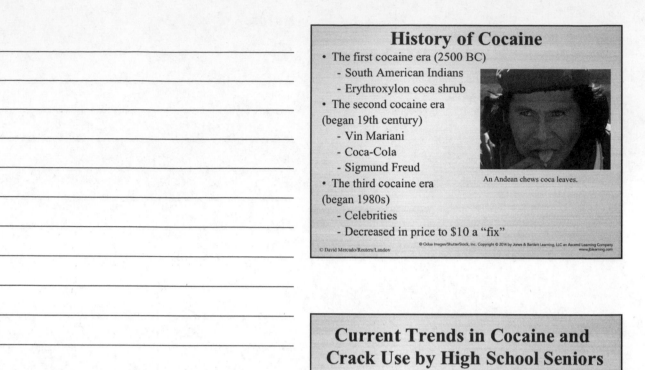

History of Cocaine

- The first cocaine era (2500 BC)
  - South American Indians
  - Erythroxylon coca shrub
- The second cocaine era (began 19th century)
  - Vin Mariani
  - Coca-Cola
  - Sigmund Freud
- The third cocaine era (began 1980s)
  - Celebrities
  - Decreased in price to $10 a "fix"

An Andean chews coca leaves.

© David Mercado/Reuters/Landov

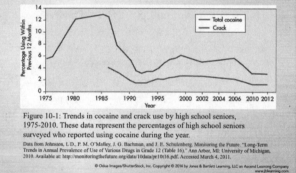

Current Trends in Cocaine and Crack Use by High School Seniors

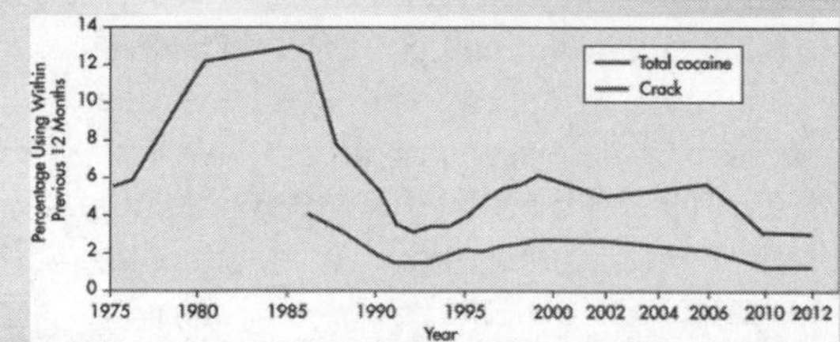

Figure 10-1: Trends in cocaine and crack use by high school seniors, 1975-2010. These data represent the percentages of high school seniors surveyed who reported using cocaine during the year.

Data from Johnston, L.D., P. M. O'Malley, J. G. Bachman, and J. E. Schulenberg. Monitoring the Future. "Long-Term Trends in Annual Prevalence of Use of Various Drugs in Grade 12 (Table 16)." Ann Arbor, MI: University of Michigan, 2010. Available at: http://monitoringthefuture.org/data/10data/pr10t16.pdf. Accessed March 4, 2011.

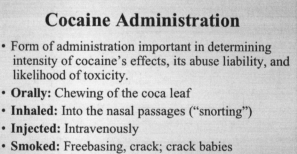

Cocaine Administration

- Form of administration important in determining intensity of cocaine's effects, its abuse liability, and likelihood of toxicity.
- **Orally:** Chewing of the coca leaf
- **Inhaled:** Into the nasal passages ("snorting")
- **Injected:** Intravenously
- **Smoked:** Freebasing, crack; crack babies

Pharmacological Effects of Cocaine

- Enhanced activity of the catecholamine and serotonin transmitters
- Blocks the reuptake of these substances following their release from neurons
- The summation of cocaine's effects on dopamine, noradrenaline, adrenaline, and serotonin is to cause CNS stimulation
  - Cardiovascular system
  - Local anesthetic effect

Main Stages of Cocaine Withdrawal

1. **Crash:** Initial abstinence phase consisting of depression, agitation, suicidal thoughts, and fatigue
2. **Withdrawal:** Including mood swings, craving, anhedonia, and obsession with drug seeking
3. **Extinction:** Normal pleasure returns, mood swings, cues trigger craving

Treatment of Cocaine Dependence

- Is highly individualistic and has variable success. Most cocaine users use other drugs as well, such as alcohol.
- Principal treatment strategies include inpatient and outpatient programs.
- Drug therapy is often used to relieve cocaine craving and mood problems.
- Psychological counseling, support, and a highly motivated patient are essential.

Notes

Notes

Cocaine and Pregnancy

- Cocaine babies; not clear the effect of cocaine on the fetus. Some possibilities are:
  - Microencephaly
  - Reduced birth weight
  - Increased irritability
  - Subtle learning and cognitive defects

Minor Stimulants

- Caffeine is the most frequently consumed stimulant in the world.
  - It is classified as a xanthine (methylxanthine)
  - It is found in a number of beverages
  - Also found in some OTC medicines and chocolate
- In the U.S., the average daily intake of caffeine is equivalent to __ cups of coffee a day.

  (Answer: 2–3)

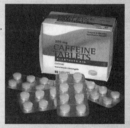

OTC caffeine products frequently contain the equivalent of 2-3 cups of coffee and are used to stay awake.

Caffeine Content of Beverages and Chocolate

Beverage	Caffeine Content (mg)/cup	Amount
Brewed coffee	90–125	5 oz.
Instant coffee	35–164	5 oz.
Decaffeinated coffee	1–6	5 oz.
Tea	25–125	5 oz.
Cocoa	5–25	5 oz.
Coca-Cola	45	12 oz.
Pepsi-Cola	38	12 oz.
Mountain Dew	54	12 oz.
Chocolate bar	1–35	1 oz.

Notes

Physiological Effects of Xanthines

- CNS effects
  - Enhances alertness, causes arousal, diminishes fatigue
- Adverse CNS effects
  - Insomnia, increase in tension, anxiety, and initiation of muscle twitches
  - Over 500 milligrams: panic sensations, chills, nausea, clumsiness
  - Extremely high doses (5 to 10 grams): seizures, respiratory failure, and death

Physiological Effects of Xanthines (continued)

- Cardiovascular effects
  - Low doses: Heart activity increases, decreases, or does nothing
  - High doses: Rate of contraction of the heart increases, minor vasodilation in most of the body, cerebral blood vessels are vasoconstricted
- Respiratory system effect
  - Can cause air passages to open and facilitate breathing

Physiological Effects of Xanthines (continued)

- Caffeine intoxication
  - Caffeinism
  - Restlessness, nervousness, excitement, insomnia, flushed face, diuresis, muscle twitching, rambling thoughts and speech, stomach complaints
- Caffeine dependence

Notes

OTC Drugs and Other Products that Contain Caffeine or Caffeine-Like Stimulants

- Analgesics
- Stay-awake products
- Picker-uppers
- Water and juices

Other Stimulants

- OTC sympathomimetics included in cold, allergic and diet aid medications
- Herbal stimulants: often contain ephedrine, ephedra, ma huang, or guarana

CHAPTER 11

Tobacco

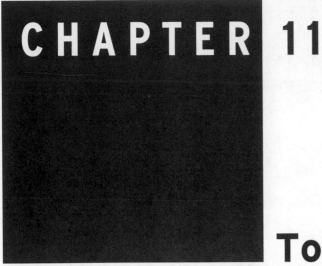

The chapter outline provides you with an organizational guide to the topics and ideas presented in this chapter of the text.

Tobacco Use: Scope of the Problem
- Current Tobacco Use in the United States
- Cigarette Smoking: A Costly Addiction

The History of Tobacco Use
- Popularity in the Western World
- History of Tobacco Use in America
- Tobacco Production
- Government Regulation

Pharmacology of Nicotine
- Effects of Nicotine on the Central Nervous System
- Other Effects of Nicotine

Cigarette Smoking
- Cardiovascular Disease
- Cancer
- Bronchopulmonary Disease
- Effects on Pregnancy

"Light" Cigarettes

Electronic Cigarettes

Tobacco Use and Exposure Without Smoking
- Smokeless Tobacco
- Secondhand Smoke

Reasons for Smoking and the Motivation to Quit
- Reasons for Smoking
- Benefits of Cessation
- The Motivation to Quit

Smoking Prohibition Versus Smokers' Rights

■ Key Terms

Define the following terms:

1. **Nicotine** ______________________________
2. **Environmental tobacco smoke** ______________________________
3. **Chewing tobacco** ______________________________
4. **Snuff** ______________________________
5. **Passive smoking** ______________________________
6. **Gateway drug** ______________________________
7. **Second-hand smoke** ______________________________
8. **Sudden Infant Death Syndrome** ______________________________

Fill-in-the-Blank

1. ______________________________ is a colorless, highly volatile liquid alkaloid.
2. ______________________________ is a finely ground tobacco that is commonly placed between the gum and cheek.
3. ______________________________ refers to a mixture of the smoke that comes directly from the tip of a lighted cigarette between puffs and smoke that has been exhaled.
4. The unexpected and unexplainable death that occurs while infants are sleeping is called ______________________________.
5. The two main forms of smokeless tobacco in the United States are ______________________________ and ______________________________.
6. ______________________________ is an antidepressant used as an aid in smoking cessation.

Identify

1. Identify three deleterious consequences of cigarette smoking.
   a. ______________________________
   b. ______________________________
   c. ______________________________
2. Identify three factors that determine the amount of nicotine absorbed into the body.
   a. ______________________________
   b. ______________________________
   c. ______________________________
3. Identify and discuss three kinds of smoking cessation aids.
   a. ______________________________
   b. ______________________________
   c. ______________________________

True/False

Tell whether each statement is true or false. If false, explain what makes the statement incorrect.

1. Tobacco use is the leading preventable cause of death in the United States. ______________________

____

2. Smoking during pregnancy does not affect the fetus. ______________________________________

____

3. There are currently no pharmacology therapies that are FDA-approved to aid in smoking cessation.

____

____

Discussion Questions

1. What efforts has the government made to decrease tobacco use? Do you think these are enough? ____

____

____

____

2. What effects do cigarettes have on the central nervous system? What other effects do cigarettes have on the body? ____

____

____

____

3. How safe are smokeless tobacco products compared with cigarettes? ___________________________

____

____

____

4. Why do people smoke? ____

____

____

____

5. Should smokers have the right to smoke in public places? Defend your answer. ____________________

____

____

____

Notes

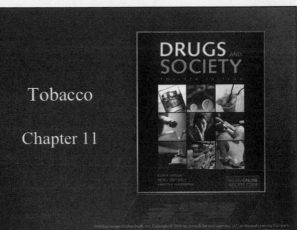

Tobacco Use: Scope of the Problem

- Tobacco use is the leading preventable cause of disease and premature death in the United States.
  - 443,000 deaths annually in United States
- Tobacco is the single largest cause of preventable death and a risk factor for 6/8 of the leading causes of death.

Current Tobacco Use in the U.S.

- In 2011, 68.2 million Americans, or 26.5% of the population age 12 or older, reported current use of a tobacco product.
- Approximately 32.3 percent of males and 21.1% of females age 12 or older were current users of any tobacco product.

Notes

Tobacco Use: A Costly Addiction

- More deaths are caused each year by tobacco use than by HIV, illegal drug use, murders, alcohol use, suicides, and motor vehicle injuries combined.

History of Tobacco Use

- Mayans: tobacco smoke as "divine incense"
- Turkey: poets vs. priests
- France: Louis XIII vs. Louis XIV
- Nicholas Monardes: infallible cure
- Pope Urban VII: excommunication for tobacco users

History of Tobacco Use in America

- Cigars became popular in the United States in the early 1800s.
- The introduction of the cigarette-rolling machine spurred cigarette consumption because cigarettes became cheaper than cigars.

Notes

Tobacco Production

- Nicotiana tabacum is the primary species of tobacco.
- Flue-cured tobacco is cured with heat transmitted through a flue without exposure to smoke or fumes.

Government Regulation

- 1964: The Advisory Committee to the U.S. Surgeon General reported that cigarette smoking is related to lung cancer.
- 1970: Warnings on cigarette labels.

Master Settlement Agreement

- Limitations on advertising
- Ban on cartoon characters in advertising
- Ban on "branded" merchandise
- Limitations on sponsoring of sporting events
- Disbanding of tobacco trade organizations
- Funds designated to support anti-smoking measures and research to reduce youth smoking

Notes

Family Smoking Prevention and Control Act

- Gave FDA authority to regulate the manufacture, distribution, and marketing of tobacco products
- Restricts cigarette sales to youth and requires proof of age

Pharmacology of Nicotine

- It is a colorless, highly volatile liquid alkaloid.
- When smoked, nicotine enters the lungs and is then absorbed into the bloodstream.
- When chewed or dipped, nicotine is absorbed through the mucous lining of the mouth.

Pharmacology of Nicotine

- Amount of tobacco absorbed depends on
  - Exact composition of tobacco
  - How densely the tobacco is packed in the cigarette
  - Whether a filter is used and characteristics of filter
  - The volume of smoke inhaled
  - The number of cigarettes smoked

Notes

Physiological Effects

- Stimulates central dopamine release
- Stimulates cardiovascular system

Cigarette Smoking

- Cigarette smokers not only tend to die at an earlier age than nonsmokers, but also have a higher probability of developing certain diseases, including cardiovascular disease, cancer, bronchopulmonary disease, and other illnesses

Cardiovascular Disease

- Smoking causes coronary heart disease, the leading cause of death in the United States.
- Compared with non-smokers, smoking increases the risk of coronary heart disease two to four times.
- Smoking puts smokers at greater risk for developing peripheral artery disease.

Notes

Cancer

- Cigarette smoking is a major cause of cancers of the lung, bladder, pancreas, cervix, esophagus, stomach, oral cavity and kidney.
- The risk of lung cancer in men who smoke two or more packs per day is 23 times greater than the risk for nonsmokers, while the risk for women is approximately 13 times greater.

Bronchopulmonary Disease

- Cigarette damages the airways and alveoli, and causes emphysema, chronic airway obstruction, and emphysema

Cigarette smoking is a leading cause of bronchopulmonary disease.

Effects on Pregnancy

- One in six pregnant women smoked cigarettes in the past month
- Increased risk for stillbirth, pre-term delivery, infertility, low birth weight and sudden infant death syndrome

Light Cigarettes

- There is no conclusive evidence of reduced health risks associated with low-tar cigarettes.
- Filtered cigarettes reduce levels of tar, nicotine, and carbon monoxide at the mouth end of the filter and should be of some limited benefit.
- Many smokers lose this benefit because they often smoke more cigarettes per day, increase puff number and volume, or block the filter holes with their fingers or lips.

Electronic Cigarettes

- Electronic cigarettes (e-cigarettes) are devices designed to deliver nicotine or other substances to a user as a vapor.
- The FDA has not evaluated e-cigarettes for effectiveness or safety.

Tobacco Use Without Smoking

- Chewing tobacco and snuff.
- Use can lead to nicotine addiction and dependence.
- Contains 28 cancer-causing agents.
- Smokeless tobacco is strongly associated with leukoplakia.
- Smokeless tobacco increases the risk of developing cancer of the oral cavity and pancreas.
- Smokeless tobacco use during pregnancy increases the risks for preeclampsia, premature birth, and low birth weight.

Notes

Notes

Secondhand Smoke

- **Secondhand smoke** includes a mixture of smoke that comes directly from the lighted tip of a cigarette, cigar, or pipe tip and exhaled smoke
- **Passive smoking** refers to nonsmokers' inhalation of tobacco smoke.
- Secondhand smoke exposure causes an estimated 46,000 heart disease deaths annually in the United States.

Benefits of Cessation

1. A return to normalcy of heart rate and blood pressure (which are abnormally high while smoking).
2. A decline of carbon monoxide in the blood within hours.
3. Improved circulation, production of less phlegm, and decreased rate of coughing and sneezing within weeks.
4. Substantial improvements in lung function within several months.

Benefits of Cessation (continued)

5. Decreased risk for lung and other types of cancer.
6. Decreased risk for coronary heart disease, stroke, and peripheral vascular disease.
7. Decreased respiratory symptoms such as coughing, wheezing, and shortness of breath.

Benefits of Cessation (continued)

8. Decreased risk of developing chronic obstructive pulmonary disease.
9. Decreased risk for infertility in women.
10. Decreased risk of having a low birth weight baby.

Methods for Quitting

- Nicotine gum
- Nicotine patches
- Nicotine spray
- Nicotine lozenges
- Bupropion
- Varenicline

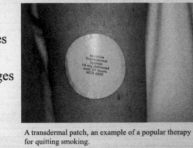

A transdermal patch, an example of a popular therapy for quitting smoking.

Notes

CHAPTER 12

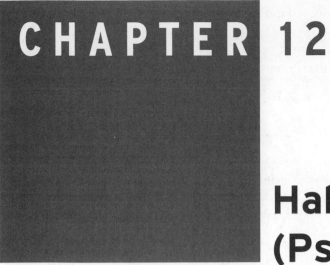

Hallucinogens (Psychedelics)

The chapter outline provides you with an organizational guide to the topics and ideas presented in this chapter of the text.

Key Terms

Define the following terms:

1. **Hallucinogens** ____________________
2. **Psychotomimetic** ____________________
3. **Synesthesia** ____________________
4. **Ergotism** ____________________
5. **Mydriasis** ____________________
6. **Entactogen** ____________________
7. **Jimsonweed** ____________________
8. **Catatonia** ____________________

Fill-in-the-Blank

1. ____________________ are substances that expand or heighten perception and consciousness.
2. Substances that initiate psychotic behavior are ____________________.

3. ______________________ are recurrences of earlier drug-induced sensory experiences in the absence of the drug.

4. ______________________ are drugs that enhance the sensation and pleasure of touching.

5. Drugs that are chemically related to amphetamines are called ______________________.

■ Identify

1. Identify the four stages of sensory experiences typically experienced by users of LSD.

   a. ______________________

   b. ______________________

   c. ______________________

   d. ______________________

2. Identify and describe three categories of negative LSD-related flashbacks.

   a. ______________________

   b. ______________________

   c. ______________________

3. What are some effects of using mescaline? ______________________

   ____

   ____

4. Briefly discuss the effects of the following hallucinogens:

   a. Psilocybin ______________________

   ____

   b. DMT ______________________

   ____

   c. Nutmeg ______________________

   ____

   d. MDMA (ecstasy) ______________________

   ____

   e. Phencyclidine (PCP) ______________________

   ____

5. Identify and briefly describe three examples of anticholinergic hallucinogens.

   a. ______________________

   b. ______________________

   c. ______________________

■ Discussion Questions

1. Should Native Americans be allowed access to otherwise illegal drugs for religious purposes? ________

2. How does LSD affect a user's behavior and perception? ________

3. What dangers does a person face if they decide to take hallucinogenic street drugs? ________

4. Why did MDMA decrease in popularity after 2002? What are some negative effects of MDMA that users should be aware of? ________

5. Why is PCP considered to be the most dangerous of hallucinogens? ________

6. What effects can be caused by abusing dextromethorphan? Should OTC products that contain this drug be placed behind the counter? ________

7. What is salvia divinorum? Should it be Scheduled? Justify your answer. ________

Notes

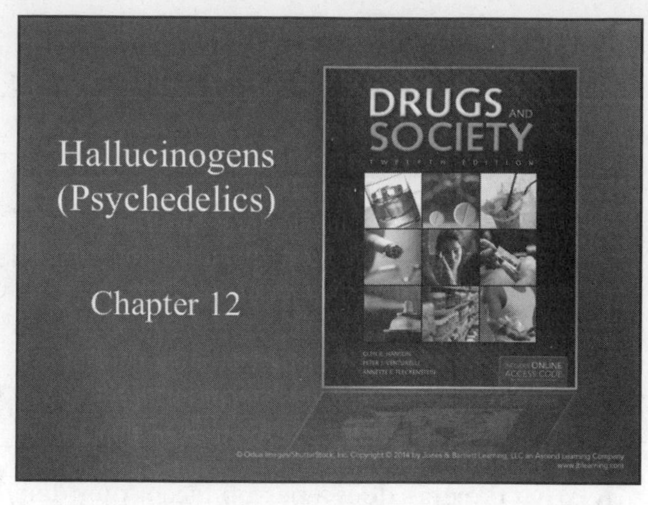

Hallucinogens

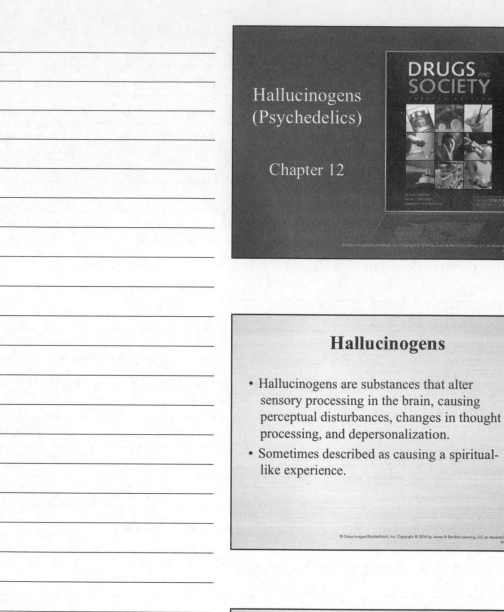

- Hallucinogens are substances that alter sensory processing in the brain, causing perceptual disturbances, changes in thought processing, and depersonalization.
- Sometimes described as causing a spiritual-like experience.

History of Hallucinogens

- The Native American Church:
  - The American Indian Religious Freedom Act of 1978
- Timothy Leary and the League of Spiritual Discovery:
  - *The Psychedelic Experience*
- Some mental health providers claim these drugs can assist with psychotherapy.

Notes

The Nature of Hallucinogens

- Many drugs can exert hallucinogenic effects:
  - Traditional hallucinogens (LSD-types)
  - Phenylethylamines (Ecstasy, amphetamines)
  - Anticholinergic agents (Jimsonweed and other natural products)
  - Cocaine
  - Steroids

Nature of Hallucinogens

- Psychedelic
- Psychotogenic
- Psychotomimetic

Sensory and Psychological Effects of Hallucinogens

- Altered senses
  - Synesthesia
- Loss of control
  - Flashbacks
- Self-reflection
  - "Make conscious the unconscious"
- Loss of identity and cosmic merging
  - "Mystical-spiritual aspect of the drug experience"

Notes

Traditional Hallucinogens: LSD Types of Agents

- LSD (lysergic acid diethylamide), mescaline, psilocybin, dimethyltryptamine (DMT), and myristicin
- These drugs cause predominantly psychedelic effects
- Of high school seniors sampled:
  - 1996: 8.8% had used LSD
  - 2012: 2.4% had used LSD

Traditional Hallucinogens: LSD Types of Agents (continued)

- Physical properties of LSD
  - In pure form: colorless, odorless, tasteless
  - Street names: acid, blotter acid, microdot, window panes
- Mechanism of action
  - Likely due to effects on the serotonin system

Traditional Hallucinogens: LSD Types of Agents (continued)

- Physiological effects:
  - Massive increase in neural activity in some brain regions ("electrical storm").
  - Activates sympathetic nervous system (rise in body temperature, heart rate, and blood pressure).
  - Parasympathetic nervous system (increase in salivation and nausea).
  - Individuals do not become physically dependent, but psychological dependency can occur.

Traditional Hallucinogens: LSD Types of Agents (continued)

- Effects of this hallucinogen begin 30–90 minutes after ingestion and can last up to 12 hours.
- Tolerance to the effects of LSD develops very quickly.
- Behavioral effects:
  - Creativity and insight
  - Adverse psychedelic effects
  - Perceptual effects

Other LSD Types of Agents

- Mescaline (Peyote)
  - Mescaline is the most active drug in peyote; it induces intensified perception of colors and euphoria.
  - Effects include dilation of the pupils, increase in body temperature, anxiety, visual hallucinations, alteration of body image, vomiting, muscular relaxation.
  - Street samples are rarely authentic.

Other LSD Types of Agents (continued)

- Psilocybin
  - Principle source is the *Psilocybe mexicana* mushroom.
  - It is not very common on the street.
  - Hallucinogenic effects similar to LSD.
  - Cross-tolerance among psilocybin, LSD, and mescaline.
  - Stimulates autonomic nervous system, dilates the pupils, increases body temperature.

Notes

Notes

Other LSD Types of Agents (continued)

- Dimethyltryptamine (DMT)
  - A short-acting hallucinogen.
  - Trace amounts are found in the body.
  - Found in seeds of certain leguminous trees and prepared synthetically.
  - It is inhaled and is similar in action to psilocybin.

Other LSD Types of Agents (continued)

- Foxy
  - Relatively new hallucinogen.
  - Lower doses: euphoria.
  - Higher doses: similar to LSD.
- Nutmeg
  - Myristica oil responsible for physical effects.
  - High doses can be quite intoxicating.
  - Often causes unpleasant trips.

Phenylethylamine Hallucinogens

- The phenylethylamine drugs are chemically related to amphetamines.
- They have varying degrees of hallucinogenic and CNS stimulant effects.
  - LSD-like: predominantly release **serotonin**; dominated by their **hallucinogenic** action.
  - Cocaine-like: predominantly release **dopamine**; dominated by their **stimulant** effects.

Phenylethylamine Hallucinogens (continued)

- Dimthoxymethylamphetamine (DOM or STP)
- "Designer" amphetamines
  - 3,4-Methylenedioxyamphetamine (MDA)
  - Methylenedioxymethamphetamine
  - (MDMA, Ecstasy); referred to as an *entactogen* (in 2012 used by 3.8% of high school seniors)

Anticholinergic Hallucinogens

- The anticholinergic hallucinogens include naturally occurring alkaloid substances that are present in plants and herbs.
- The potato family of plants contains most of these mind-altering drugs.
- Three potent anticholingergic compounds in these plants:
  - Scopolamine
  - Hyoscyamine
  - Atropine

Naturally Occurring Anticholinergic Hallucinogens

- *Atropa Belladonna*: The Deadly Nightshade
- *Mandragora Officinarum:* The Mandrake
- *Hyoscyamus Niger:* Henbane
- *Datura Stramonium:* Jimsonweed

Notes

Notes

Other Hallucinogens

- Phencyclidine (PCP)
  - Considered by many experts as the most dangerous of the hallucinogens although it has a host of other effects as well.
  - It was developed as an intravenous anesthetic but was found to have serious adverse side effects.

Other Hallucinogens (continued)

- Phencyclidine (PCP) physiological effects
  - Hallucinogenic effects, stimulation, depression, anesthesia, analgesia
  - Large doses can cause coma, convulsions, and death
- PCP psychological effects
  - Feelings of strength, power, invulnerability, perceptual distortions, paranoia, violence, and psychoses and users appear like schizophrenics

Other Hallucinogens (continued)

- Ketamine (general anesthetic; PCP-like)
- Dextromethorphan (cough suppressant)
  - High doses cause PCP-like effects
  - Commonly abuse by adolescents (5.6% high school seniors used in 2012)
- Marijuana
- *Salvia divinorum*
  - "Legal" hallucinogenic herb, used by 4.4% of high school seniors in 2012
  - Can cause intense hallucinations and short-term memory loss

CHAPTER 13

Marijuana

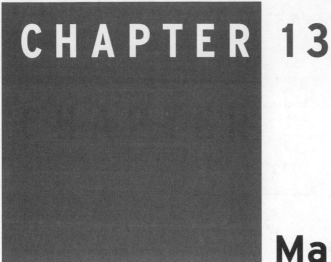

The chapter outline provides you with an organizational guide to the topics and ideas presented in this chapter of the text.

Introduction
Marijuana: History and Current Trends
- Historical Roots of Marijuana
- Current Use of Marijuana
- Recent Trends in Use of Marijuana: 8th, 10th, and 12th Graders

Marijuana: Is it the Assassin of Youth?
- Major Factors Affecting Marijuana Use

Is Marijuana Really a Gateway Drug?
- Misperceptions of Marijuana Use
- Characteristics of Cannabis

The Behavioral Effects of Marijuana Use
- The High
- Subjective Euphoric Effects
- Driving Performance
- Critical Thinking Skills
- Amotivational Syndrome

Therapeutic Uses and the Controversy over Medical Marijuana Use
- Reduction in Intraocular (Eye) Pressure
- Antiasthmatic Effect
- Muscle-Relaxant Effect
- Antiseizure Effect
- Antidepressant Effect
- Analgesic Effect
- Antinauseant
- Appetite Stimulant

Short-Term Dangers of Smoking Marijuana
Long-Term Consequences of Smoking Marijuana
The Physiological Effects of Marijuana Use
- Effects on the Brain
- Effects on the Central Nervous System
- Effects on the Respiratory System: Smoking Marijuana
- Effects on the Respiratory System: Vaporizing Marijuana
- Effects on the Cardiovascular System
- Effects on Sexual Performance and Reproduction
- Tolerance and Dependence
- Chronic Use

Key Terms

Define the following terms:

1. *Cannabis sativa* ______________________
2. *Cannabis indica* ______________________
3. Gateway drugs ______________________
4. Hashish ______________________

5. **Subjective euphoric effects** ______________________________

____

6. **Differential association** ______________________________

7. **Amotivational syndrome** ______________________________

8. **Glaucoma** ______________________________

9. **Altered perceptions** ______________________________

10. **Anandamide** ______________________________

■ Fill-in-the-Blank

1. ____________________ are complex illegal organizations that produce, transport, and/or distribute large quantities of one or more illicit drugs.

2. Meaning without seeds, ____________________ is made from the buds and flowering tops of female plants and is one of the most potent types of marijuana.

3. ____________________ involves using the THC in cannabis as a drug to calm or to relieve symptoms of an illness.

4. Hunger experienced while under the effects of marijuana is called the ____________________.

5. A compound that is believed to be the cause of sexual arousal is an ____________________.

6. Recently, instead of smoking marijuana, some have resorted to ____________________, which involves heating cannabis to high temperatures to release cannabinoids in a fine mist.

■ Identify

1. Identify three possible medical uses of marijuana.

a. ______________________________

b. ______________________________

c. ______________________________

2. Identify three short-term dangers of marijuana use.

a. ______________________________

b. ______________________________

c. ______________________________

3. Describe the effects of marijuana on the following systems:

a. Central nervous system ______________________________

____

b. Respiratory system ______________________________

____

c. Cardiovascular system ______________________________

____

■ Discussion Questions

1. Do you believe that prosecution for marijuana possession should be more or less rigid than it currently is? Why? ______________________________

____

____

____

2. Debate whether marijuana use adversely affects driving capabilities. ______________________________

____

____

____

3. Why is marijuana attractive to many individuals? ______________________________

____

____

____

4. Should marijuana be legalized for medical use? Defend your answer. ______________________________

____

____

____

Notes

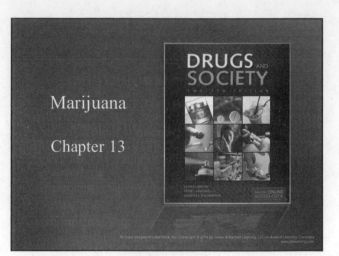

What Is Marijuana?

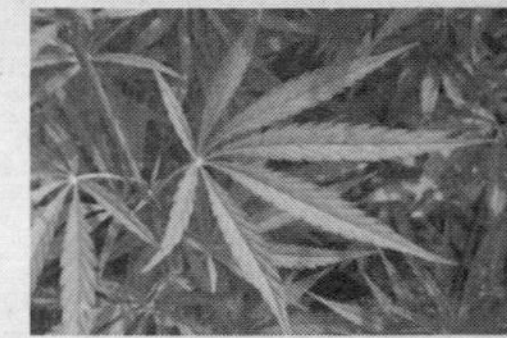

- **Marijuana** is a hemp plant whose biological name is *cannabis sativa*. It consists of green, brown, or a grey mixture of dried, shredded leaves, stems, seeds, and flowers.
- **THC** (delta-9-tetrahydrocannabinol) is the primary mind-altering ingredient in marijuana.

© stdesign/Shutterstock, Inc.

Brief History and Trends

- Marijuana has historically been a valued crop. The woody fibers of the stem yield a fiber that can be made into cloth and rope.
- Early records of marijuana use:
  - China 2737 BC and India (religious ceremonies)
  - Assyrians, dating back to 650 BC used it for making rope, cloth, and consumed it to experience euphoria
  - Ancient Greeks also knew about marijuana
  - In North America, in Jamestown (1611), marijuana was used to make rope and clothing
  - Currently, marijuana grows wild in many U.S. states

Notes

Several Questions and Answers

- *Today marijuana is how many times more potent than the marijuana on the street in the 1960s and 1970s?*
  - Approximately 20 times more potent as result of more efficient agriculture largely due to new methods of harvesting, new varieties, and special processing marijuana of plants

Several Questions and Answers (continued)

- *How many Americans are current marijuana users?*
  - Aged 12 or older in 2011: Out of 18.1 million illicit drug users, *approximately* 64.3% reported *current use* of only marijuana and another 16.2% used marijuana with another illicit drug. (This means that a staggering 80.5% [64.3% + 16.2%] either used marijuana alone or used marijuana with another drug.) The remaining 19.5% of drug users used an illicit drug but not marijuana.

Noteworthy Findings Regarding Marijuana Users

- It is the most highly abused illicit type of illicit drug.
- The highest rate of use was found among young adults (ages 18–25) with 18.9% reporting current use (past month) and among youth (ages 12–17) with 7.6% reporting current use.
- The average age of first use was 17.5 years.
- There were 2.6 million new marijuana users in 2011, which averages 7,200 initiates per day.

Notes

Major Factors Affecting Marijuana Use

- **Structural factors:** Age, gender, family background, lack of any religious beliefs
- **Social and interactional factors:** Type of interpersonal relationships, friendship cliques, drug use within the peer group setting
- **Setting:** Type of community and neighborhood (physical location of drug use)
- **Attitudinal factors:** Personal attitudes toward the use of drugs, self esteem, maturation level

Major Factors Affecting Marijuana Use (continued)

- **Participation in after-school activities** is associated with higher levels of academic achievement and self-esteem, as well as lower levels of substance use
- **Religious involvement** affects illicit drug use and this clearly includes marijuana use

Cannabis Use Disorder Defined by DSM-V*

- *Cannabis* is often taken in larger amounts than was intended
- There are persistent desires or unsuccessful efforts to cut down or control *cannabis* use
- Much time is spent securing the drug, using the drug and/or recovering from its effects
- Craving the euphoric effects of the drug
- Failure to fulfill major role obligations at work, school, or home
- Continued use of *cannabis* despite persistent or recurrent social and interpersonal problems cased by the effect of cannabis

Cannabis Use Disorder Defined by DSM-V* (continued)

- Important social, occupational or recreational activities are given up or reduced because of *cannabis* use
- Recurrent *cannabis* usage in situations in which it is physically hazardous
- *Cannabis* use is continued despite persistent or recurrent physical or psychological problems stemming from usage
- Tolerance develops to offset the diminishing effects of cannabis resulting in more use of *cannabis*
- Withdrawal symptoms lead to increased use of cannabis

*These two slides, (slides 9 and 10), are Heavily paraphrased from American Psychiatric Association (APA). "Substance-Related and Addictive Disorders." In *Diagnostic and Statistical Manual of Mental Disorders (DSM-5)*, 5th ed., 509–510. Arlington, VA: American Psychiatric Association, 2013.

Marijuana

- **Gateway drugs** are drugs that often lead to the use of more addictive types of drugs (gateway to the use and abuse of other more potent drugs).
  - Alcohol, tobacco, and marijuana are the drugs most commonly believed to be gateway drugs.
  - Other common gateway drugs include inhalants and anabolic steroids. More recently, the abuse of prescription drugs (mainly painkillers) are also included.

Two Major Types of Marijuana

- ***Cannabis Sativa:***
  - Originates from Colombia, Mexico, Jamaica, South Africa, Thailand, and Southeast Asia
  - Causes uplifting and energetic feelings, appetite stimulant, and provides pain relief
- ***Cannabis Indica:***
  - Originates from hash producing with very warm climates in such countries Afghanistan, Pakistan, India, Turkey, Morocco, and Tibet
  - Causes body relaxation, stress relief, and calmness and serenity and has lower THC content than *Sativa*

Notes

Notes

Varieties of Marijuana from the *Cannabis Sativa* Plant

- **Hashish:** Average concentration of THC is 12.1% for domestic, 7.03% for non-domestic, and 20.76 for samples seized by law enforcement officials
- **Ganja:** Consists of the dried tops of female plants. The term is also used as a slang term for marijuana (pot, weed, reefer)
- ***Sinsemilla*** (without seeds), **"hydro"** (grown in water), **kind bud**, **dro**, **30s**, **AK-47**, and **blueberry** (more recent names of popular types of marijuana). The average concentration of THC is 7.5% and higher
- **Bhang:** Average concentration of THC is 1% to 2%

Behavioral Effects

- Low to moderate doses produce euphoria and a pleasant state of relaxation.
- Common effects: dry mouth, elevated heartbeat, some loss of coordination and balance, slower reaction times, reddening of the eyes, elevated blood pressure, some mental confusion (short-term memory loss).
- A typical high lasts from 2 to 3 hours (length of effect depends on amount of THC), and the user experiences altered perception of space and time as well as impaired memory.

Behavioral Effects (continued)

- An acute dose of cannabis can produce adverse reactions: mild anxiety to panic and paranoia.
- In a minority of cases users can exhibit psychosis, delusional and bizarre behavior, and hallucinations. These reactions occur most frequently in individuals who are under stress, anxious, depressed, or borderline schizophrenic, and are using the more potent types of marijuana.

Notes

Behavioral Effects (continued)

- **Subjective euphoric effects:** The ongoing social and psychological experiences incurred while intoxicated with marijuana. These include both the user's altered state of consciousness and his/her perceptions while intoxicated.
- **Attachment to the use of Marijuana**: Users exhibit a strong attachment to their passsionate feelings about using marijuana.
- **Differential association:** Behavioral satisfaction derived from friends who use marijuana ("fun-times when high with friends").

Driving Performance

- The ability to perform complex tasks, such as driving, is often impaired while under the influence of marijuana.
- In limited surveys, from 70% to 80% of marijuana users indicate that they sometimes drive while being high.
- Research reveals that approximately 600,000 high school seniors drive after smoking marijuana (DEA, 2006) and 41% of teens were not concerned about driving after taking drugs. (Driving while under the influence of a drug termed **drugged driving**.)
- Habitual cannabis users were 9.5 times more likely to be involved in crashes.

Critical Thinking Skills

- Marijuana has been found to have a negative impact on critical thinking skills.
- Specifically, heavy marijuana use impairs attention, memory and learning.
- Marijuana alters brain activity because residues of this drug persist in the brain.

Notes

Amotivational Syndrome or Anti-motivational Syndrome

- **Amotivational syndrome** refers to a belief that heavy use of marijuana causes a lack of motivation or impaired desire and reduced productivity.
- Specifically, users show an increase in:
  - Apathy
  - Poor short-term memory
  - Difficulty with concentration
  - A lingering lack of interest in pursuing goals

Therapeutic Uses of Marijuana

- **Medical marijuana use:** Involves using the THC derived from smoking marijuana or using Marinol as a drug to calm or relieve symptoms of an illness. (Marinol is an FDA-approved THC in capsule form.)
- Some research shows that THC can be used for treating:
  - Glaucoma: potentially blinding eye disease causing continual and increasing intraocular pressure

Therapeutic Uses of Marijuana (continued)

- **Appetite stimulant:** Patients experiencing anorexia, AIDS, chemotherapy and radiation therapy
- **Antiseizure:** Aids in the prevention of seizures (epilepsy)
- **Antiasthmatic effect:** Short-term smoking of marijuana improves breathing for asthma patients
- **Antidepressant effect:** Used in Great Britain as a euphoriant for treating depression
- **Muscle relaxation:** Aids in reducing muscle spasms
- **Analgesic effect:** In patients experiencing frequent migraines and chronic headaches or inflammation

Arguments Against Marijuana Use

- It contains 421 chemicals.
- It is stronger than it was 20 years ago.
- Smoking this drug is worse for the lungs than tobacco.
- Impairs short-term memory and may cause "amotivational syndrome."
- U.S. federal law continues to legally prohibit the possession, the sale, and use of marijuana. (The federal government believes marijuana has no medically proven use.)

Physiological Effects

- **The brain:** THC activates the reward system in the brain by stimulating brain cells to release the chemical dopamine
- **Central nervous system:** Alters mood, coordination, memory, and self-perception
- **Respiratory system:** Damage to the lungs
- **Cardiovascular system:** Marijuana products limit the amount of oxygen that can be carried to the heart
- **Sexual performance and reproduction:** Affects the sympathetic nervous system, increasing vasodilation in the genital and delaying ejaculation; high doses can decrease sexual desire

Effects of Marijuana on the Central Nervous System

- **Altered perceptions**
  - Changes in the interpretation of stimuli resulting from marijuana use
- **"Munchies"**
  - Hunger experienced while under the effects of marijuana
- **Anandamide**
  - Possible neurotransmitter acting at the marijuana (cannabinoid) receptor site

Notes

Notes

Effects on Other Systems

- **Alveolar Macrophages** (respiratory system)
  - Special white blood cells that play a role in cleaning lung tissue are less able to remove debris when exposed to smoke
- **Vasodilation** (cardiovascular system)
  - Enlarged blood vessels
- **Aphrodisiac** (sexual performance and reproduction)
  - In lower doses of marijuana, THC is believed to cause sexual arousal

CHAPTER 14

Inhalants

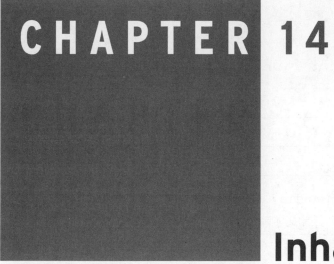

The chapter outline provides you with an organizational guide to the topics and ideas presented in this chapter of the text.

Introduction
History of Inhalants
Types of Inhalants
- Volatile Substances
- Anesthetics
- Nitrites

Legislation
Current Patterns and Signs of Abuse
- Adolescent and Teenage Usage
- Gender, Race, Socioeconomics, and Abuse
- Signs of Inhalant Abuse

Dangers of Inhalant Abuse

Key Terms

Define the following terms:

1. **Volatile** ______________________________
2. **Euphorigenic** ______________________________
3. **Arrhythmia** ______________________________
4. **Hypoxia** ______________________________

Fill-in-the-Blank

1. An irregular heartbeat is called an ______________________________.
2. ______________________________ is a state of oxygen deficiency.
3. Gasoline is an example of a ______________________ substance and is abused commonly by young people due to its widespread availability.

■ Identify

1. Give four signs of inhalant abuse.

a. ______________________________

b. ______________________________

c. ______________________________

d. ______________________________

2. Name four of the many products misused as inhalants today.

a. ______________________________

b. ______________________________

c. ______________________________

d. ______________________________

3. Identify and discuss the three major groups of inhalants.

a. ______________________________

b. ______________________________

c. ______________________________

■ Discussion Questions

1. Why are inhalants popular? Give several reasons. ______________________________

____

____

____

2. Why is inhalant abuse such a serious problem? What are the dangers and misconceptions associated with inhalant abuse? ______________________________

____

____

____

Notes

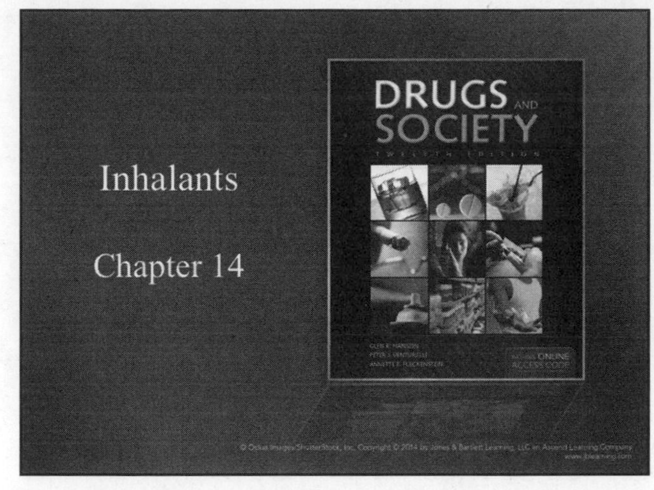
Inhalants
Chapter 14
DRUGS AND SOCIETY

Introduction

- Volatile substances introduced via the lungs.
- Most cause intoxicating and/or euphorigenic effects.
- Many of these substances were never intended to be used by humans as drugs; consequently, they are not often thought of as having abuse potential.

Introduction (continued)

- Inhalants are among the most commonly used drugs by adolescents.
- A widespread misconception is that inhalant abuse is a harmless phase that occurs commonly during normal childhood and teenage development and as such is not worthy of significant concern.

Notes

Potential Consequences

- "Sudden Sniffing Death Syndrome" (SSDS): A condition characterized by serious cardiac arrhythmia occurring during or immediately after inhaling
- Brain damage
- Damage to heart, kidney, liver, and bone marrow

Considerations

- Synergistic effects
- Lipid (fat) composition
- Developmentally immature users

History

- In 1776, British chemist Joseph Priestley synthesized nitrous oxide, a colorless gas with a slightly sweet odor and no noticeable taste.
- Priestly and Humphry Davy suggested correctly that the gas might be useful as an anesthetic, and experiments were conducted to test this possibility.

History (continued)

- Abuse of inhalants came to public attention in the 1950s when the news media reported that young people were getting high from sniffing glue.

Legislation

- Inhalants are generally not regulated as are other drugs of abuse.
- Some states have adopted laws preventing the use, sale, and/or distribution to minors of various products abused commonly as inhalants.

Types of Inhalants

- Volatile substances
- Anesthetics
- Nitrites

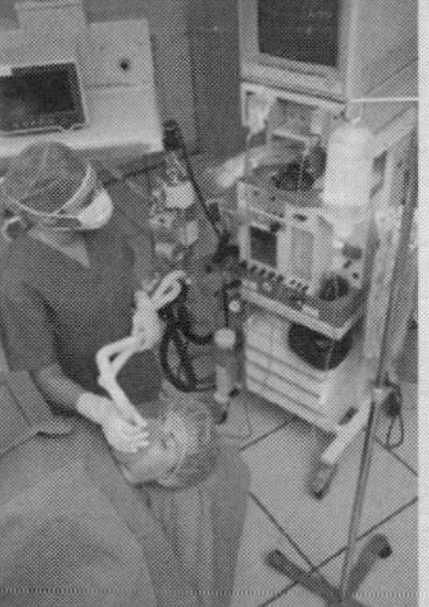

Anesthetics are an example of an inhalant.

Notes

Notes

Volatile Substances

- Includes aerosols, art or office supplies, adhesives, fuels, and industrial or household solvents.
- Some abusers inhale vapors directly from their original containers (called sniffing or snorting).
- Some abusers inhale volatile solvents from plastic bags (called bagging) or from old rags or bandannas soaked in the solvent fluid and held over the mouth (called huffing).

Potential Effects of Inhaling Volatile Substances

- Can cause irritation of airways causing coughing and sneezing.
- Low doses often bring a brief feeling of lightheadedness, mild stimulation followed by a loss of control, lack of coordination, and disorientation accompanied by dizziness and possible hallucinations.
- In some instances, higher doses can produce relaxation, sleep or even coma.

Potential Effects of Inhaling Volatile Substances (continued)

- If inhalation is continued, dangerous hypoxia may occur and cause brain damage or death.
- Other effects include hypertension and damage to the cardiac muscle, peripheral nerves, brain, and kidneys.
- Chronic abusers of inhalants frequently lose their appetite, are continually tired, and experience nosebleeds.

Aerosols

- Include spray paints, deodorant and hair sprays, vegetable oil sprays for cooking, and fabric protector sprays
- Often abused not because of the effects produced by their principal ingredients but rather because of the effects of their propellant gases
- Can be dangerous because these devices are capable of generating very high concentrations of the inhaled chemicals

Toluene

- Found in some glues, paints, thinners, nail polishes, and typewriter correction fluid
- A principal ingredient in "Texas shoe shine"
- Detectable in the arterial blood within 10 seconds of inhalation exposure
- Highly lipid soluble
- Can cause brain damage, impaired cognition and gait disturbances
- Liver and kidney damage have been reported

Butane and Propane

- Found commonly in found in lighter fluid, hair and paint sprays.
- SSDS, and serious burn injuries (because of flammability) have resulted from abuse

Notes

Notes

Gasoline

- A mixture of volatile chemicals, including toluene, benzene, and triorthocresyl phosphate (TCP)
- Because of its widespread availability, young people, particularly in rural settings, sometimes abuse gasoline

Gasoline (continued)

- As a mixture of chemicals, its intentional inhalation can be especially dangerous.
  - Benzene is an organic compound that causes impaired immunologic function, bone marrow injury, increased risk of leukemia, and reproductive system toxicity.
  - TCP is a fuel additive that causes degeneration of motor neurons.

Freons

- Freons and other related agents are used in refrigerators, air conditioners, and airbrushes.
- Inhalation can cause not only serious liver damage but also SSDS.
- Inhalation can cause freeze injuries.

Anesthetics (e.g. Nitrous Oxide)

- "Laughing gas": frequently used in outpatient procedures
- Can also be sold in large balloons or small cylindrical cartridges used as charges for whipped cream dispensers

Nitrous Oxide

- Significant abuse problems of nitrous oxide are infrequent, but there are occasional reports of severe hypoxia or death due to acute overdoses
- Can cause loss of sensation, limb spasms, altered perception and motor coordination, blackouts resulting from blood pressure changes and reduced cardiac function.

Nitrites

- Cause vasodilation
- Prototype, amyl nitrite, has been used in the past to treat angina
- Abuse has decreased dramatically

Notes

Notes

Why Abused?

- Legally obtained
- Readily available
- Inexpensive
- Easy to conceal
- Lack of information about potential dangers

Who Abuses?

- Primarily adolescents, but even small children.
- More adolescent males than females.
- Chronic inhalant users frequently have a profile like that associated with other substance abusers. That is, often they live in unhappy surroundings with severe family or school problems, they have poor self-images, and sniffing gives them an accessible escape.

Signs of Inhalant Abuse

- Often collect an unusual assortment of chemicals (such as glues, paints, thinners and solvents, nail polish, liquid eraser, and cleaning fluids) in bedrooms or with belongings
- Have breath that occasionally smells of solvents
- Often have the sniffles similar to a cold but without other symptoms of the ailment

Signs of Inhalant Abuse (continued)

- Appear drunk for short periods of time (15 to 60 minutes) but recover quickly
- Do not do well in school and are usually unkempt
- Sitting with a pen or marker near nose
- Constantly smelling clothing sleeves

Signs of Inhalant Abuse (continued)

- Hiding rags, clothes, or empty containers of the potentially abused products in closets, boxes, and other places
- Possessing chemical-soaked rags, bags, or socks
- Abusable household items missing

Dangers of Inhalants

- Sudden sniffing death syndrome
- Damage to brain, liver, kidney, heart
- Choking on vomit
- Accidents associated with "intoxication" and fires

Notes

CHAPTER 15

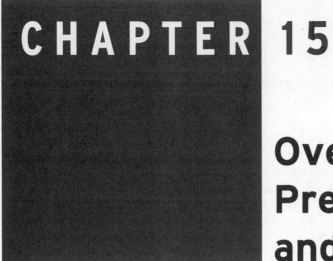

Over-the-Counter, Prescription, and Herbal Drugs

The chapter outline provides you with an organizational guide to the topics and ideas presented in this chapter of the text.

Key Terms

Define the following terms:

1. **Analgesics** ______________________________
2. **Salicylates** ______________________________
3. **Anti-inflammatory** ______________________________
4. **NSAIDs** ______________________________
5. **Congestion rebound** ______________________________
6. **Gastritis** ______________________________
7. **Keratolytics** ______________________________
8. **SPF number** ______________________________
9. **Monoamine oxidase inhibitors (MAOIs)** ______________________________
10. **Diabetes mellitus** ______________________________
11. **Peptic ulcers** ______________________________

12. **Hypertension** ______________________________

13. **Ischemia** ______________________________

14. **Angina pectoris** ______________________________

15. **Edema** ______________________________

■ Fill-in-the-Blank

1. ______________________ are potent hormones released from the adrenal glands.
2. Drugs that reduce fevers are ______________________.
3. ______________________ is a potentially fatal complication of colds, flu, or chicken pox in children.
4. Drugs that block the coughing reflex are ______________________.
5. Substances that stimulate mucous secretion and diminish mucous viscosity are ______________________.
6. ______________________ are drugs that suppress the activity of the brain's appetite center, causing reduced food intake.
7. The outermost protective layer of the skin is the ______________________.
8. The most commonly used group of drugs to treat severe depression is ______________________.
9. Drugs taken by mouth to treat type II diabetes are ______________________.
10. Drugs that widen air passages are called ______________________.
11. ______________________ occurs when the heart is unable to pump sufficient blood for the body's needs.
12. ______________________ occurs when the thyroid gland does not produce sufficient hormones.

■ Identify

1. Identify six kinds of information that must appear on the labels of an OTC medicinal product.

a. ______

b. ______

c. ______

d. ______

e. ______

f. ______

2. Identify three types of drugs used to treat the common cold. Indicate the symptoms for which each drug is used.

a. ______

b. ______

c. ______

3. Identify three common over-the-counter drugs and their uses.

a. ______

b. ______

c. ______

4. Identify the criteria, according to the Durham-Humphrey Amendment of 1951, to determine if a drug should be controlled with prescriptions.

a. ______

b. ______

c. ______

d. ______

5. Give five reasons why prescription drug abuse occurs.

a. ______

b. ______

c. ______

d. ______

e. ______

6. Identify five signs of patients with drug-seeking behavior.

a. ______

b. ______

c. ______

d. ______

e. ______

7. Identify three common categories of prescription drugs and explain their uses.

a. ______

b. ______

c. ______

True/False

Tell whether the statement is true or false. If false, explain what makes the statement incorrect.

1. OTC drugs are always safe and effective for consumer use. ______

______

2. Abuse of prescription drugs is almost always less dangerous than abuse of illegal drugs. ______

______

Discussion Questions

1. What are some concerns about the FDA's switching policy? Do you think switching prescription drugs to OTC status is a safe decision? Defend your answer. ______

______

______

______

2. Why does abuse of OTC products often occur? ______

______

______

______

3. What rules should be followed to ensure safe OTC drug use? ______

______

______

______

4. What regulation is placed on OTC herbal products? Should there be more? Are these products safe? __

5. Why is it important to communicate with your doctor? What questions should you ask to ensure that you are being given appropriate prescriptions? ______

6. Why has abuse of prescription drugs become such a problem for our society? ______

7. How do generic drugs compare to proprietary ones? ______

8. What is the difference between type I and type II diabetes? ______

Notes

Over-the-Counter, Prescription, and Herbal Drugs

Chapter 15

DRUGS AND SOCIETY

Prescription and OTC Drugs

- **Prescription** drugs are available only by recommendation of a licensed health professional, such as a physician.
- **Nonprescription** (over-the-counter, or OTC) drugs are available on request and generally do not require approval by a health professional.

Prescription and OTC Drugs (continued)

- Prescription and OTC drugs have been viewed differently by the public since the classifications were established by the Durham-Humphrey Amendment of 1951.
- In general, the public views OTC drugs as less effective, safe, and rarely abused and prescription drugs as more potent and potentially dangerous. However, these distinctions are not always accurate.

OTC Drugs Interesting Facts

- Each year, people in the United States spend over $18 billion on OTC drugs.
- More than 100,000 different OTC products are available on the market.
- OTC expenditures comprise 60% of the annual drug purchases in the United States.
- An estimated 60.6% people routinely self-medicate with these drug products.

Abuse of OTC Drugs

- OTC products generally have a greater margin of safety than their prescription counterparts, but issues of abuse need to be considered.
- Physical dependence.
- Psychological dependence.

Abuse of OTC Drugs (continued)

- Nonprescription products that can be quite habit-forming: decongestants, laxatives, antihistamines, sleep aids, and antacids.
- OTC drugs are more likely to be abused by members of the general public who inadvertently become dependent due to excessive self-medication than by hardcore drug addicts.

Notes

Notes

"Switching" Policy of the FDA

- The FDA is attempting to make more drugs available to the general public by switching some frequently used and safe prescription medications to OTC status.
- There have been approximately 90 active ingredients switched, leading to hundreds of new OTC drug products.

OTC Drugs and Self-Care

- Many of the major health problems in the United States can be treated with OTC medications.
- If done correctly, self-care with OTC medications can provide significant relief from minor, self-limiting health problems at minimal cost.

OTC Labels

- Required label information includes:
  - Approved uses of the product
  - Detailed instructions on safe and effective use
  - Cautions or warnings to those at greatest risk when taking the medication

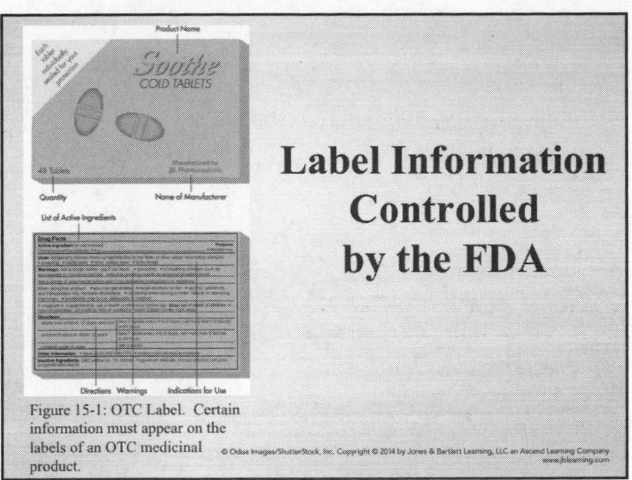

Figure 15-1: OTC Label. Certain information must appear on the labels of an OTC medicinal product.

Notes

Rules for Proper OTC Drug Use

- Always know what you are taking.
- Know the effects.
- Read and heed the warnings and cautions.
- Don't use anything for more than 1 to 2 weeks.
- Be particularly cautious if also taking prescription drugs or herbal products.
- If you have questions, ask a pharmacist.
- If you don't need it, don't use it!

Types of OTC Drugs

- Internal analgesics
  - Salicylates
  - Acetaminophen
  - Ibuprofen
  - Ibuprofen-like
- Therapeutic considerations
  - Analgesic actions
  - Anti-inflammatory effects
  - Antipyretic effects
  - Side effects

Notes

Types of OTC Drugs (continued)

- Cold, allergy, and cough remedies
  - Decongestants
  - Antitussives
  - Expectorants
- Sleep aids
  - Antihistamines
  - Melatonin
- Stimulants
  - Stay-awake or energy-promoting

Types of OTC Drugs (continued)

- Gastrointestinal medication
  - Antacids and anti-heartburn medication
- Diet aids
- Skin products
  - Acne medications
  - Sun products
- Skin first-aid products
- OTC herbal products

Prescription Drugs

- There are currently more than 10,000 prescription products sold in the United States, representing:
  - Approximately 1500 different drugs
  - With 20 to 50 new medications approved each year by the FDA
- 3.9 billion drug prescriptions were written in 2009 at a cost of ~$300 billion

Prescription Drugs (continued)

- According to the Durham-Humphrey Amendment of 1951, drugs are controlled with prescription if they are:
  - Habit-forming
  - Not safe for self-medication
  - Intended to treat ailments that require the supervision of a health professional
  - New and without an established safe track record

Prescription Drug Abuse

- Overall cost of prescription painkiller abuse is $70 billion per year
- There are more than 40 deaths from prescription painkillers in the US annually
- There have been a 4-fold increase in incidents of prescription abuse in the last 10 years
- 70% of those who abuse prescription drugs get them from friends and relations

Prescription Drug Abuse (continued)

- Illicit use of prescription drugs may be prompted by several reasons, such as:
  - To relieve withdrawal caused by drug habits
  - To treat infections caused by drug abuse
  - To provide a source of fresh, clean needles for injecting drugs of abuse
  - To prolong high caused by other drugs of abuse

Notes

Notes

Doctor–Patient Communication

- When a physician prescribes a drug, a patient should insist on answers to the following questions:
  - What is being treated?
  - What is the desired outcome?
  - What are the possible side effects of the drug?
  - How should the drug be taken to minimize problems and maximize benefits?

In order to maximize benefit and minimize risk, there must be proper doctor-patient communication.

© LiquidLibrary

Generic Versus Proprietary Drugs

- **Generic:** The official, nonpatented, nonproprietary name of a drug. The term *generic* is used by the public to refer to the common name of a drug that is not subject to trademark rights.
- **Proprietary:** A brand or trademark name that is registered with the U.S. Patent Office. Proprietary denoted medications are marketed under specific brand names, such as Valium.

Common Categories of Prescription Drugs

- Analgesics
  - Nonsteroidal anti-inflammatory (NSAIDS)
  - Narcotic analgesics
- Antibiotics
  - Antibacterials
- Antidepressants
- Antidiabetic drugs
- Antiulcer drugs
- Bronchodilators

Common Categories of Prescription Drugs (continued)

- Cardiovascular drugs
  - Antihypertensive agents
  - Antianginal agents
  - Drugs to treat congestive heart failure
  - Cholesterol and lipid-lowering drugs
- Hormone-related drugs
- Sedative-hypnotic agents
- Stimulants
- Drugs to treat HIV

Common Principles of Drug Use

- Patients should ask the following:
  - Why am I taking this drug?
  - How should I be taking this drug?
  - What are the active ingredients?
  - What are the most likely side effects?
  - How long should I be taking this drug?

How to Deal With Unused Prescription Drugs

- Do not flush extra medications, it may contaminate the water
- Store in a secure place so they can't be stolen
- Do not leave labels with your personal information on prescription drugs you are disposing
- Place drugs in bag with either coffee or cat litter before throwing it away
- Drop medications off at a secure drop off box

Notes

CHAPTER 16

Drug Use in Subcultures of Special Populations

The chapter outline provides you with an organizational guide to the topics and ideas presented in this chapter of the text.

Introduction
Athletes and Drug Abuse
- Laws Intended to Stop the Use of Performance-Enhancing Drugs in Professional Sports
- Drugs Used by Athletes
- Prevention and Treatment

Drug Use Among Women
- Women More Concerned About Drug Use than Men
- Patterns of Drug Use: Comparing Females with Males
- Female Roles, Seeking Treatment, and Drug Addiction
- Women's Response to Drugs
- Treatment of Drug Dependence in Women
- Prevention of Drug Dependence in Women

Drug Use in Adolescent Subcultures
- Consequences of Underage Drug Use
- Why Adolescents Use Drugs
- Patterns of Drug Use in Adolescent Families
- Current Changes in Teen Drug Use Cause Concern
- Adolescent Versus Adult Drug Abuse
- Consequences and Coincidental Problems
- Prevention, Intervention, and Treatment of Adolescent Drug Problems
- Summary of Adolescent Drug Abuse

Drug Use in College Student Subcultures
- Reasons for College Students' Drug Use
- Additional Noteworthy Findings Regarding Drug Use by College Students
- Recommendations for Reducing Drug Use and Abuse on College Campuses

HIV and AIDS
- Major U.S. Statistics and Trends in Specific Populations Living with HIV/AIDS
- Nature of HIV Infection and Related Symptoms
- Diagnosis and Treatment
- Who Is at Risk for AIDS?
- AIDS and Drugs of Abuse
- Youth and AIDS
- What to Do About HIV and AIDS

The Entertainment Industry and Drug Use
Promoters of Drug Use: The Internet

Key Terms

Define the following terms:

1. **Subculture** ____________________
2. **Outsider's perspective** ____________________
3. **Insider's perspective** ____________________

4. **World Anti-Doping Code** ______________________________

5. **Ergogenic** ______________________________

6. **Anabolic steroids** ______________________________

7. **Muscle dysmorphia** ______________________________

8. **Cycling** ______________________________

9. **Pyramiding** ______________________________

10. **Human growth factor** ______________________________

11. **Sociobiological changes** ______________________________

12. **Rohypnol** ______________________________

13. **Protease inhibitors** ______________________________

14. **Highly active antiretroviral therapy (HAART)** ______________________________

____

■ Fill-in-the-Blank

1. Using performance-enhancing drugs to increase athletic ability is called ____________________.

2. ____________________ are naturally occurring male hormones, such as testosterone.

3. Use of several types of steroids at the same time is called ______________________________

   ____________________.

4. ____________________ involves developing a tolerance to the effects of anabolic steroids.

5. The use of other drugs while taking anabolic steroids to avoid possible side effects is known as an _____

   ______________________________.

6. A "designer drug" synthetic version of human growth factor (HGF) is ______________________________

   ____________________.

7. ____________________ is the drug most widely used and abused by women in the United States.

8. ____________________ violence occurs between members of the same gang, while ____________________ occurs between members of different gangs.

■ Identify

1. Why would individuals within various subcultures initially turn to drugs? Provide three internal subculture forces and three external subculture forces.

Internal Subculture Forces

a. ______

b. ______

c. ______

External Subculture Forces

a. ______

b. ______

c. ______

2. Identify four possible adverse effects of heavy steroid use.

a. ______

b. ______

c. ______

d. ______

3. What attracts adolescents to gangs? Identify five things that gangs offer often troubled adolescents.

a. ______

b. ______

c. ______

d. ______

e. ______

4. How can one prevent adolescent gang involvement? Offer three suggestions.

a. ______

b. ______

c. ______

5. Identify five behaviors that act as warning signs that adolescents may be abusing drugs.

a. ______

b. ______

c. ______

d. ______

e. ______

■ Discussion Questions

1. Why do athletes often risk using drugs?

2. What is the ATLAS program? Is this program an effective tool for the prevention of steroid use by athletes?

3. How do the roles of females in society affect their drug use?

4. Why are women less likely than men to seek treatment for, and rehabilitation from, drug dependence?

5. Why do adolescents use drugs?

6. How are patterns of drug use in adolescents different from drug use patterns in adults?

7. How does drug use contribute to teen suicide?

8. Why do college students use drugs? ______________________________

____

____

____

9. How does AIDS relate to drug abuse? ______________________________

____

____

____

10. How does the entertainment industry affect drug use? ______________________________

____

____

____

11. In what ways does the Internet promote drug use? ______________________________

____

____

____

Notes

Drug Use in Subcultures of Special Populations

Chapter 16

DRUGS AND SOCIETY

TWELFTH EDITION

Subcultures of Special Populations

- Athletes/those involved in sports
- Women
- Adolescents
- College Students
- HIV and AIDS Carriers
- Promoters of Drug Use: The Entertainment Industry and the Internet

Subculture

- A **subculture** is defined as a special population or subgroup whose members share similar values and patterns of related behaviors that differ from the larger population.
- Two types of factors that function as forces affecting members of a drug-using subculture are:
  - **Internal subcultural forces:** Shared attitudes that are favorable of drug use, habitual, and/or addictive behavior
  - **External subcultural forces:** Law enforcement, availability of drug dealers, and concerns with being caught using drugs

Two Major Perspectives

- **Outsider's Perspective**
  - Viewing a group or subculture from outside the group and viewing the group and its members as an observer; looking "in." Non-users viewing drug-users.
- **Insider's Perspective**
  - Viewing a group or subculture from inside the group; seeing members as they perceive themselves. Drug users in agreement with other drug users or sympathizers.

Athletes and Drug Abuse

- Drug abuse has been reported since the Greeks started the Olympics in 776 BC.
- "Doping" among world-class competitors is rampant.
- Young athletes often receive exaggerated attention and prestige in almost every university, college, high school, and junior high school in the United States.

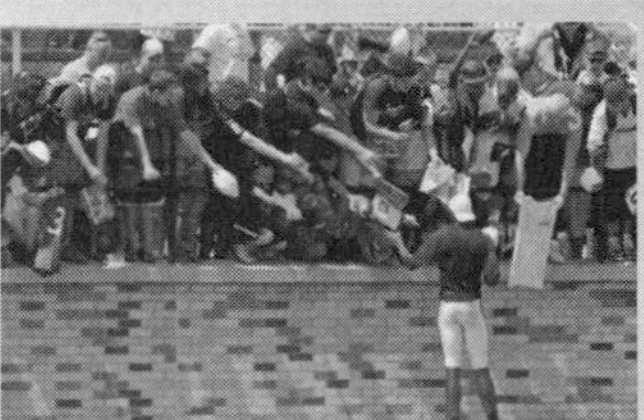

Besides risking their health, athletes who choose to dope should remember that they are role models. Seventy-three percent of youth want to be like a famous athlete; 53% of youth say it is common for famous athletes to use banned substances to get ahead.

Athletes and Drug Abuse (continued)

- Studies have shown that athletes are *not* more likely than non-athletes to use drugs of abuse such as marijuana, alcohol, barbiturates, cocaine, and hallucinogens.
- However, *athletes are much more likely than other subcultures of drug users to take drugs to enhance performance*. These drugs include stimulants such as amphetamines, cocaine, and an array of drugs with presumed ergogenic effects, such as anabolic steroids.

Notes

Notes

Drugs Used by Athletes

- **Anabolic steroids** consist of a group of natural and synthetic drugs that are chemically similar to cholesterol and related to the male hormone testosterone.
- Naturally occurring male hormones, or **androgens**, are produced by the testes in males.

The Most Commonly Abused Steroids

- **Oral Steroids:**
  - Anadrol (oxymetholone), Oxandrin (oxandrolone), Dianabol (methandrostenolone), and Winstrol (stanozolol)
- **Injectable Steroids:**
  - Deca-Durabolin (nandrolone decanoate), Durabolin (nandrolone phenpropionate), Depo-Testosterone (testosterone cypionate), Equipoise (boldenone undecylenate), and Tetrahydrogestrinone (THG)

Major Reasons for the Use/Abuse of Anabolic Steroids

- Improve athletic performance.
- Increase muscle size or reduce body fat.
- Experienced physical or sexual abuse (e.g., female weightlifters who had been raped were found to be twice as like to use anabolic steroids).

Major Reasons for the Use/Abuse of Anabolic Steroids (continued)

- Adolescent steroid abusers often take risks such as drinking and driving, carrying a gun, driving a motorcycle without a helmet, and abusing other types of illicit drugs.
- Muscle dysmorphia, is a behavioral syndrome that causes individuals to have a distorted image of their bodies (i.e., perceiving themselves as looking small and weak, even when they may be large and muscular), may be a reason to use anabolic steroids.

Abuse of Anabolic Steroids by Athletes

- Under some conditions, androgen-like drugs can increase muscle mass and strength.
- An estimated 1 million Americans have used or are using these drugs to achieve a "competitive edge."
  - Males are much more likely to use steroids than females.
  - 1.3% of 8th graders and 10th graders and 2.2% of 12th graders had used steroids during their lifetimes.
  - Among seniors in high school, 3.2% males and 1.1% females used steroids while 1.5% of college-aged men used.

Extent of Steroid Usage in Professional Sports

- Usage patterns for anabolic steroids vary considerably according to athletes' motivation, level of competition, the type of sport, and the pressure for winning.
- "Of the 26 sports included in the 2012 Games, the worst offender in terms of the rate of findings per sample (averaged across all eight years) is cycling, 3.71%."
- "The second highest rate - 3.05% - was found among boxers. Badminton had the lowest rate of usage-indication findings per sample, at 0.87%."
- "Footballers were the most tested athletes in terms of the total number of samples (30,398), followed by athletics (25,013), cycling (21,427) and aquatics (13,138)" (*Guardian* [The] 2012).

Notes

Notes

Patterns of Anabolic Steroid Use by Athletes

- **Stacking:** Use of several types of steroids at the same time.
- **Cycling:** Use of different steroids taken singly but in sequence.
- **Plateauing:** Developing tolerance to a particular steroid.
- **Pyramiding:** Beginning steroid use with low doses moving to higher doses, then reducing the dosage at the end of the cycle.
- **Array:** Use of other drugs while taking anabolic steroids to avoid possible side effects, such as taking diuretics, anti-acne, anti-estrogens.

Effects of Anabolic Steroids

- Increased strength
- Increased lean body mass
- Increased "bad" blood cholesterol
- Increased risk of liver disorders
- Psychological effects: irritability, outbursts of anger like "road rage," mania, psychosis, and major depression
- Psychological and physical dependence with continual use of high doses

Effects of Anabolic Steroids (continued)

- Withdrawal symptoms: craving, fatigue, depression, restlessness, loss of appetite, insomnia, diminished sex drive, headaches
- Alterations in reproductive systems and sex hormones:
  - Breast enlargement in males; breast reduction and hair growth in females
  - Infertility
  - Atrophy (shrinkage of the penis and testicles in males and enlargement of external genitalia in females)

Effects of Anabolic Steroids (continued)

- Stunted growth in adolescents
- Deepening of voice in females
- Water retention
- Change in skin and hair (severe acne, male pattern baldness, and increased body hair)
- Persistent unpleasant breath odor
- Swelling of feet and limbs

Drugs Used by Athletes

- Stimulants (amphetamines and cocaine)
- Clenbuterol
- Erythropoietin
- Human growth factor (HGF) and human growth hormone (HGH)
- ß-adrenergic blockers
- Gamma-hydroxybutyrate

Drug Use Among Women with Comparisons to Men (1975-2011)

- Overall, females consistently use fewer licit and illicit drugs: 31.3% of females versus 36.6% of males use illicit drugs
- Most types of abused drugs by females (in descending order):
  - Alcohol, females 83.1% (males 84.7%)
  - Flavored alcoholic beverages, females 60.2% (males 46.5%)
  - Binge drinking (+5 or more drinks) in last two weeks, females 29% (males 45.4%)
  - Cigarettes, females 27.8% (males 35.9%)
  - Marijuana, females 26.3% (males 34.1%)
  - Any illicit drug other than marijuana, females 15.6% (males 19.2%)

Notes

Notes

Drug Use Among Women with Comparisons to Men (1975-2011) (continued)

- Narcotics other than heroin, females 7.2% (males 8.6%)
- Amphetamines, females 5.8% (males 7.7%)
- Cocaine, females 3.3% (males 6.4%)
- Hallucinogens, females, 2.2% (males 5.3%)
- Hallucinogens other than LSD, females 1.7% (males 4.7%)

- Steroids, females 0.1% (males 0.3%
- Finally, nationwide surveys confirm that drug use is often increasing among women more rapidly than among men (Drug Strategies, 1998; NSDUH, 2007).

How Do These Drugs Affect a Woman's Reproduction?

- Cocaine? A substantial threat to the fetus
- Alcohol? Crosses the placenta and affects the fetus' s development
- Tobacco? Twenty percent of pregnant females smoke cigarettes. (May be greater threat to the fetus than cocaine.)
- Other drugs (marijuana, LSD, other depressant drugs)? Associated with abnormal fetal development when used during pregnancy

Women and Alcohol

- Alcohol is the drug most widely used and abused by women in the United States.
  - Women aged 12 and older: 45.9% used alcohol in the past month and 15.2% reported binge drinking.
  - Unlike men, women are less likely to develop severe alcohol dependence (only 25% of the alcoholics in the United States are female).
- Women dependent on alcohol are judged more harshly than men dependent on alcohol.

Why Adolescents Use Drugs

- Most adolescents who use substances of abuse during psychosocial development do not develop problematic drug dependence.
- Adolescent users who have difficulty with drugs often lack coping skills, are from dysfunctional families, maintain poor self-images, and/or feel socially and emotionally insecure.

Why Adolescents Use Drugs (continued)

- Parents who are most likely to foster drug abusing children are:
  - Drug abusers themselves
  - Excessively rigid and condemning *or* range from intermittent extreme rigidity to extreme neglect
  - Overly demanding
  - Overly protective
  - Overwhelmed with their own personal conflicts
  - Unable to effectively communicate with their children

Why Adolescents Use Drugs (continued)

- Recent research indicates that the most important factor influencing drug use among adolescents is peer drug use.
- Research also shows that there exists a correlation between strong family bonds and non-drug–using peer groups.
- Use drugs to cope with boredom, unpleasant feelings, emotions, and stress or to relieve depression, reduce tension, and reduce alienation.

What other explanations not mentioned above can you offer that may explain why adolescents use drugs?

Notes

Notes

Patterns of Drug Use in 8th Graders

- Fill in the blanks regarding recent surveys on lifetime drug patterns of 8th graders in 2012.
  A. __% had used alcohol
  B. __% had used cigarettes
  C. __% had used inhalants
  D. __% had used marijuana

Key: A is 29.5%, B is 15.5%, C is 11.8%, and D is 15.2%.

Patterns of Drug Use in 12th Graders

- Fill in the blanks regarding recent surveys (2012) on lifetime drug patterns of 12th graders.
  A. __% had used alcohol
  B. __% had used cigarettes
  C. __% had used inhalants
  D. __% had used marijuana

Key: A is 69.4%, B is 39.5%, C is 7.9%, and D is 45.2%.

Most Common Sources for Adolescents Obtaining Prescription Drugs

- "Given for free by a friend or relative" (51%)
- "Bought from a friend or relative" (35%)
- "Taking the drug from a friend or relative without asking" (12%)
- "Bought prescription drug on the Internet" (2%)

Notes

Past Year Adolescent Initiates of Prescription Drug Use

- In 2006, more than 2.1 million teens abused drugs
- In 2011 an average of 35% of 8th, 10th, and 12th graders used an illicit drug during their lifetime.
- Every day, 2500 youth (12–17) abuse a prescription pain reliever for the very first time.
- One-third of all new abusers of prescription drugs in 2006 were 12- to 17-year-olds.
- Prescription drugs are the drug of choice among 12- to 13-year-olds.
- Pain relievers like Vicodin and OxyContin are the prescription drugs most commonly abused by teens.

Past Year Adolescent Initiates of Prescription Drug Use (continued)

- The prescription drugs most commonly abused by teens are painkillers, powerful narcotics prescribed to treat pain; depressants, such as sleeping pills or anti-anxiety drugs; and stimulants, mainly prescribed to treat attention-deficit hyperactivity disorder (ADHD).
- Among teens who have abused painkillers, nearly one-fifth (18%) used them at least weekly in the past year.

Adolescent Drug Use: Additional Recent Findings (Johnston et al. 2012a)

- **Alcohol Use:**
  - Nearly three out of every four 12th-grade students (72%) have tried alcohol
  - Two-fifths (43%) are current drinkers
  - 8th graders – two-fifths (39%) reported some alcohol use, and one-sixth (16%) are current (past-30-day) drinkers.
  - 18% of 8th graders, 37% of 10th graders, and 54.2 of 12th graders indicated they have been drunk at least once in their lifetime and drank alcohol to the point of inebriation

Notes

Adolescent Drug Use: Additional Recent Findings (Johnston et al. 2012a) (continued)

- **Cigarettes:**
  - Nearly half (45%) of 12th graders reported having tried cigarettes
  - One-fifth (20%) smoked at least some cigarettes in the prior 30 days
  - Daily use of cigarettes in the prior 30 days of have been surveyed is considerably higher for cigarettes than for marijuana or alcohol

Consequences of Adolescent Drug Use

- Adolescent suicide
- Sexual violence and drugs
- Gangs and drugs

Prevention and Treatment of Adolescent Drug Problems

- Encourage parental awareness of gangs.
- Encourage alternative participation in organizations or groups (athletics, school activities, career development, or involvement in volunteering programs).
- Help children to develop coping skills regarding frustration and stress.
- Educate children about gang-related problems and help them understand that like drugs, gangs are the result of problems and are not the solutions to problems.

Drug Use by College Students

- Most popular substance of use and abuse is alcohol (77.4% of college students).
- 36.3% of college students report use of illicit drugs
- 33.2% report use of marijuana (Johnston et. al, 2012)
- College students who frequently binge drink are more likely to smoke cigarettes and use illegal drugs as well.
- A clear relationship exists between alcohol use and grade point average (GPA). (The more alcohol consumed the lower the GPA.)

Drug Use by College Students (continued)

- "Nearly 80% of binge drinkers live in a fraternity or sorority house, often off campus" (Marklein, 2000).
- Almost *half* of college students who were victims of campus crimes said they were drinking or using other drugs when they were victimized.
- Researchers estimate that alcohol use is implicated in one- to two-thirds of sexual assault and acquaintance or date rape cases among teens and college students.

Drug Use by College Students (continued)

- In 2011, college students were modestly higher in annual and 30-day use of alcohol than the same-aged noncollege group (often referred to as others); the difference was largest in the 30-day rate (64% vs. 56%)
- 36% of college students binged on alcohol versus 32% of the noncollege group
- Full-time college students were slightly less likely to use any illicit drugs in 2011 than the noncollege group (36% versus 39%) (Johnston et. al. 2012)
- Whites are highest binge drinkers followed by blacks and then Asians.

Notes

Notes

Drug Use by College Students (continued)

- High percentage of drinkers (approximately 50%) had altercations with law enforcement officials while consuming extraordinary amounts of alcohol.
- Other results showed that alcohol use was associated with serious and acute problems such as alcoholism, poor academic performance, drinking and driving, and criminalistic behavior (e.g., driving while intoxicated, vandalism, violence).

Drug Use by College Students (continued)

- The amount and proportion of alcohol consumed by college students varies depending on where they live.
  - Drinking rates are highest in fraternities and sororities followed by on-campus housing (e.g., dormitories, residence halls).
  - Students who live independently off-site (e.g., in apartments) drink less, while commuting students who live with their families drink the least.

Drug Use by College Students (continued)

- Fill in the blanks regarding recent surveys on annual drug patterns of full-time college students

A. ___% had used alcohol
D. ___% had used marijuana
C. ___% had used cigarettes
D. ___% had used any illicit drug
E. ___% had used amphetamines

Key: A is 77.4%, B is 33.2%, C is 25.8%,
D is 16.8%, and E is 9.3%.

Summary Findings: Drug Use and College Students from 2008-2011

- **Drugs Declining in Use:** alcohol, cigarettes, hallucinogens, methamphetamine, cocaine, sedatives (barbiturates), inhalants, and heroin
- **Drugs holding relatively steady:** Any illicit drug, any illicit drug other than marijuana, marijuana, LSD, Adderall, Crystal Methamphetamine (ice), crack, narcotics (other than heroin), OxyContin, Vicodin, and tranquilizers

Summary Findings: Drug Use and College Students from 2008-2011 (continued)

- **Drugs *increasing* in use:** Any illicit drug; alcohol; marijuana; amphetamines; cocaine; tranquilizers; sedatives (barbiturates); inhalants; heroin; rohypnol; GHB; and ketamine

Major Reasons Cited by College Students for Their Drug Use*

- Breaks the ice (74.4%)
- Enhances social activity (74.4%)
- Gives people something to do (71.7%)
- Gives people something to talk about (66.5%)
- Allows people to have more fun (63.1)
- Facilitates connections with peers (61.7%)
- Facilitates male bonding (60.1%)
- Facilitates sexual opportunity (53%)
- Facilitates female bonding (51.7)
- Makes it easier to deal with stress (43.9%)

* Sample survey of 48,650 total students with 38% male and 62% female college students and their use of alcohol and other drugs (SIUCC/Core Institute 2013).

Notes

Notes

Nature and Extent of HIV Infection and Related Symptoms (AIDS)

- Estimates are that throughout the world 33.4 million are currently living with HIV/AIDS (AIDS.gov 2012a).
- More than 25 million people have died of AIDS worldwide since the first cases were reported in 1981 (AIDS.gov 2012)
- In the United States, "CDC (Centers for Disease Control) estimates that 1,148,200 persons aged 13 years and older are living with HIV infection, including 207,600 (18.1%) who are unaware of their infection" (CDC 2012).
- Despite increases in the total number of people living with HIV in the United States in recent years, the annual number of new infections has remained relatively stable.

Nature and Extent of HIV Infection and Related Symptoms (AIDS) (continued)

- However, HIV infections continue at far too high a level, with approximately 50,000 Americans becoming newly infected with HIV each year. On average, that's one new infection every 9.5 minutes.
- More than 15,000 people with AIDS still die each year in the United States.
- Individuals infected through heterosexual contact account for 25% of annual new HIV infections and 27% of people living with HIV.

Nature and Extent of HIV Infection and Related Symptoms (AIDS) (continued)

- While blacks represent approximately 14% of the U.S. population, the latest CDC estimates show that they account for almost half of all new infections in the United States each year (44%) as well as almost half of all people living with HIV (44%).
- Gay, bisexual, and other men who have sex with men (MSM) of all races and ethnicities remain the population most profoundly affected by HIV (CDC 2013a).

Nature and Extent of HIV Infection and Related Symptoms (AIDS) (continued)

- Estimated New HIV Infections, 2010, by Transmission Category (CDC 2013)
  - Male-to-Male Sexual Contact 63%
  - Heterosexual Contact 25%
  - Injection Drug Use 8%
  - Male-to-Male Sexual Contact and Injection Drug Use 3%
  - Other 1%

Nature and Extent of HIV Infection and Related Symptoms (AIDS) (continued)

- Approximate Percentages of AIDS Cases in Adult Women by Risk Exposure, 2010 (CDC 2013)
  - Injection Drug Use 73%
  - Heterosexual Contact 25%
  - Other 2%

Nature and Extent of HIV Infection and Related Symptoms (AIDS) (continued)

- Although males who have sex with males (MSM) represent about 4% of the male population in the United States, in 2010, MSM accounted for 78% of new HIV infections among males and 63% of all new infections. MSM accounted for 52% of all people living with HIV infection in 2009, the most recent year these data are available.
- While blacks represent approximately 14% of the U.S. population, the latest CDC estimates show that they account for almost half of all new infections in the United States each year (44%) as well as almost half of all people living with HIV (44%).

Notes

Notes

Nature and Extent of HIV Infection and Related Symptoms (AIDS) (continued)

- The rate of new HIV infections for black men is more than six times as high as that of white men, and more than two times that of Hispanic men and of black women
- Comparing 2008 to 2010, new HIV infections among black women decreased 21% (from 7,700 to 6,100); however, black women account for the vast majority (64%) of all new infections among women overall and the HIV incidence rate for black women remains 20 times as high as that of white women, and almost five times that of Hispanic women.

Nature and Extent of HIV Infection and Related Symptoms (AIDS) (continued)

- The rate of new HIV infections among Hispanic men is almost three times that of white men, and the rate among Hispanic women is more than four times that of white women.
- The most common ways women get HIV (in order) are having sex with a man who has HIV and sharing injection drug works (e.g., needles, syringes) used by someone with HIV.

Important Notes About HIV Symptoms

An HIV-infected individual may not manifest symptoms of AIDS for as many as 10 to 12 years after the initial infection. Although the HIV-infected individual may experience no symptoms, he or she is highly contagious.

Important Notes About HIV Symptoms (continued)

After an individual has become infected, he or she may have a brief flu-like illness usually within 6 to 12 weeks. It is not known what determines the length of the latency period, when symptoms are not present. The asymptomatic period eventually ends, however, and signs of immune disorder appear. Initial symptoms of this disease include night sweats, swollen lymph glands, fever, and/or headaches. Medications used to treat HIV infection (antiretroviral drugs) help many people with HIV to lower the levels of virus in their blood (viral load) to undetectable levels.

Current Major Treatments for HIV

- Protease inhibitors
- Reverse transcriptase inhibitors: nucleoside/nucleotide reverse transcriptase inhibitors (NRTIs) and non-nucleoside reverse transcriptase inhibitors (NNRTIs)
- Highly active antiretroviral therapy (HAART) (medications that are also used to treat HIV/AIDS-infected individuals)
- Integrase inhibitors: most recent medications

Two Quick Quiz Questions

- What are the approximate percentages of AIDS cases in men from the following:
  A. __ % men having sex with men
  B. __ % heterosexual contact
  C. __ % injection drug users
  D. __ % male to male sexual contact and injection drug use
  Key: A is 63%, B is 25%, C is 8%, and D is 3%
- What are the approximate percentages of AIDS cases in adult women from the following:
  A. __ % injection drug use
  B. __ % heterosexual contact
  C. __ % other
  Key: A is 73%, B is 25%, and C is 2%

Notes

Notes

Most Important Drug Use Factors for the Spread of HIV/AIDS in the U.S.

- Intravenous drug use of heroin, cocaine, or both: most important factor for the spread of HIV/AIDS
- Crack: encourages high-risk sexual activities

Youths and AIDS

- Male adolescents between the ages of 13–19 and young adult males (20-24 yearrs of age who were diagnosed with AIDS contracted the disease in the following ways (CDC 2013c):
  - Male-to-male sexual contact (91.8%)
  - Heterosexual contact (4%)
  - Male-to-male sexual contact and injection drug use (2.7%)
  - Injection drug use (IDU) (1.5%)

Youths and AIDS (continued)

- Regarding race and ethnicity, this reported group was comprised of the following
  - Males (62%) and females (64% were black/African American
  - Males (19%) and females (18%) were of Hispanic/Latino
  - Males (16%) and females (14%) were of white descent
  - Males (2%) and females (2%) were from multiple races (CDC 2013)
- Three of the principal ways adolescents become infected with HIV are as follows: (1) high-risk sexual activity (unprotected sexual intercourse is reported by more than half of adolescents by the age of 17 years); (2) injection of substances of abuse; and (3) sex with multiple partners.

Youths and AIDS (continued)

- African Americans were disproportionately affected by HIV infection, accounting for 55% of all HIV infections reported among persons aged 13–24.
- "It is estimated that 50% of all new HIV infections are among young people (about 7,000 young people become infected every day), and that 30% of the 40 million people living with HIV/AIDS are in the 15–24 age group" (World Health Organization [WHO], 2000–2004).

Youths and AIDS (continued)

- Most 13- to 19-year-old females reported contracting HIV followed by AIDS through heterosexual contact (66%), injection drug use (19%), and other/not identified causes (15%).
- Worldwide, sexual intercourse is by far the most common mode of HIV transmission.
- Most 13- to 19-year-old females reported contracting HIV followed by AIDS through heterosexual contact (66%), injection drug use (19%), and other/not identified causes (15%).

Youths and AIDS (continued)

- HIV is spreading at alarming rates among younger urban gay males who are too young to recall the beginning of the AIDS epidemic two decades ago.

Notes

Notes

Drug Use in the Entertainment Industry

- Alcohol appeared in 93% of movies, 17% of songs; tobacco appeared in 89% of movies.
- "About one-third of hit songs—including three-quarters of rap songs—have some form of explicit reference to drug, alcohol or tobacco use . . ." (Yahoo! News 2008).
- In movies depicting illicit drugs, marijuana appeared most frequently (51%); hallucinogens, heroin and other opiates, and miscellaneous others (each 12%); and crack cocaine (2%).

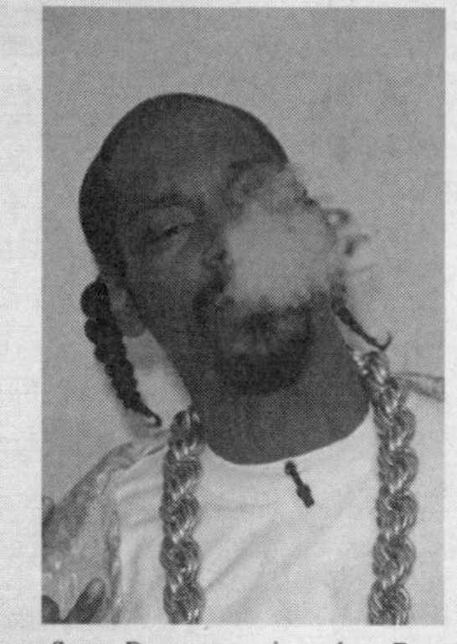

Snoop Dogg consuming a drug. Do such pictures have any effect on viewers?

Drug Use in the Entertainment Industry

Promoters of Drug Use: The Entertainment Industry and the Internet

- The Internet maintains a unique subculture of drug enthusiasts.
- Numerous web sites are used by a growing number of drug users as forums for learning and exchanging the latest information and techniques about drug use (i.e., purchasing equipment for growing, chat rooms sharing information about the use of illicit drugs, news about drug "get togethers," such as parties, raves, festival locations where drugs are prevalent).

Promoters of Drug Use: The Entertainment Industry and the Internet (continued)

- The Internet is a more recent source for marketing illicit drugs for anyone having access to computers, and this audience includes younger teens and adults. Legal suppliers appear to be fueling the trade by providing their products to unlicensed Internet pharmacies that then sell these legally restricted types of drugs (Join Together Online and BBC News 2005).

Promoters of Drug Use: The Entertainment Industry and the Internet (continued)

- The potential impact of acquiring illicit drugs from Internet sites was emphasized by a journalist warning that we should "Forget the drug dealer on the corner, teens are increasingly turning to the Internet to get high" (Fiore 2008).

Notes

CHAPTER 17

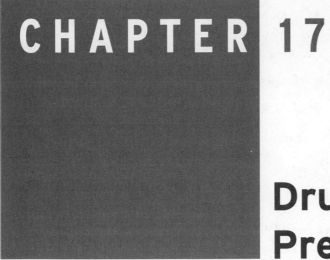

Drug Abuse Prevention

The chapter outline provides you with an organizational guide to the topics and ideas presented in this chapter of the text.

Introduction
How Serious Is the Problem of Drug Dependence?
Drug Prevention
Risk Factors and Protective Factors
Considering the Audience and Approach
Prevention Research: Key Findings
- An Example of Drug Prevention at Central High in Elmtown

Comprehensive Prevention Programs for Drug Use and Abuse
- Harm Reduction Model
- Community-Based Drug Prevention
- School-Based Drug Prevention
- Family-Based Prevention Programs
- Individual-Based Drug Prevention and Treatment: Harm Reduction Psychotherapy

Drug Prevention Programs in Higher Education
- Overview and Critique of Existing Prevention Programs

Examples of Large-Scale Drug Prevention Programs
- The BACCHUS Peer Education Network
- Fund for the Improvement of Postsecondary Education Drug Prevention Programs
- Drug Abuse Resistance Education (D.A.R.E.)
- Drug Courts

Problems with Assessing the Success of Drug Prevention Programs
Other Viable Alternatives to Drug Use
- Meditation
- The Natural Mind Approach

■ Key Terms

Define the following terms:

1. **AOD** ______________________
2. **Protective factors** ______________________
3. **Primary drug prevention programs** ______________________
4. **Secondary drug prevention programs** ______________________
5. **Tertiary drug prevention programs** ______________________
6. **Scare tactic approach** ______________________
7. **Alternatives approach** ______________________

Fill-in-the-Blank

1. The ______________________________ is a national and international association of college and university peer education programs focused on alcohol abuse prevention and other related student health and safety issues.
2. A ______________________________ is a court designed to focus on treatment programs and options in place of punishment for drug offenders.
3. ______________________________ emphasizes the exploration of positive alternatives to drug abuse by replacing the pleasurable feelings from drug use with involvement in social and educational activities.
4. ______________________________ is a state of consciousness in which there is a constant level of awareness focusing on one object.

Identify

1. Identify the three levels of drug prevention programs and indicate the audience at which each is aimed.
   a. ______________________________
   b. ______________________________
   c. ______________________________
2. Identify five categories of drug users.
   a. ______________________________
   b. ______________________________
   c. ______________________________
   d. ______________________________
   e. ______________________________
3. Identify three family-based protective factors that can insulate against drug use.
   a. ______________________________
   b. ______________________________
   c. ______________________________
4. Identify and describe four models of drug prevention in higher education.
   a. ______________________________
   b. ______________________________
   c. ______________________________
   d. ______________________________

■ Discussion Questions

1. How do school-based drug prevention programs attempt to prevent drug abuse? What topics and questions do they address? What tactics do they employ? Are these programs effective? ____________

2. What do family-based drug prevention programs need to do in order to effectively prevent drug use?

3. How can student peers be involved in helping to prevent drug use on college campuses? ____________

4. Has the DARE program been effective in preventing drug use? Explain. ____________

5. How do drug courts differ from criminal courts? How are drug users processed through drug courts? ____________

Notes

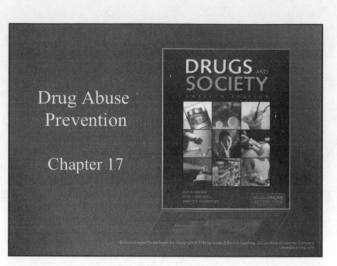

How Serious Is the Problem of Drug Dependence?

- In 2011, an estimated 20.6 million persons aged 12 or older were classified with substance dependence or abuse in the past year (8.0% of the population aged 12 or older).
- Marijuana was the illicit drug with the highest rate of past year dependence or abuse in 2011, followed by pain relievers and cocaine (highest to lowest).

How Serious Is the Problem of Drug Dependence? (continued)

- In 2011, among persons aged 12 or older, the rate of substance dependence or abuse was the lowest among Asians (3.3%). Other racial/ethnic groups with substance dependence rates included American Indians or Alaska Natives (16.8%), Native Hawaiians or Other Pacific Islander (10.6%), persons reporting two or more races (9%), Hispanics (8.7%), whites (8.2%), and blacks (7.2%).

How Serious Is the Problem of Drug Dependence? (continued)

- Rates of substance dependence or abuse were associated with *level of education* in 2011. Among adults aged 18 or older, those who graduated from a college or university had a lower rate of dependence or abuse (6.4%) than those who graduated from high school (8.0%), those who did not graduate from high school (9.3%), and those with some college (9.5%).

How Serious Is the Problem of Drug Dependence? (continued)

- Rates of substance dependence or abuse were associated with *age*. In 2011, the rate of substance dependence or abuse among adults aged 18 to 25 (18.6%) was higher than that among youths aged 12 to 17 (6.9%) and among adults aged 26 or older (6.3%).

How Serious Is the Problem of Drug Dependence? (continued)

- The rate of alcohol dependence or abuse among youths aged 12 to 17 was 3.8% in 2011, which declined from 4.6% in 2010 and from 5.9% in 2002. Among young adults aged 18 to 25, the rate of alcohol dependence or abuse also decreased between 2010 (15.7%) and 2011 (14.4%) and between 2002 (17.7%) and 2011.
- About half of the adults aged 18 or older with substance dependence or abuse were employed full time in 2011. Of the 18.9 million adults classified with dependence or abuse, 9.8 million (51.8%) were employed full time.

Notes

Notes

Goals of Prevention Programs

- Enhance protective factors (such as self-control, parental monitoring, anti-drug use policies) and reverse or reduce risk factors (such as aggressive behavior, lack of parental supervision, lure of gang membership, drug availability, and poverty).
- Address all forms of drug abuse (underage, young adult, mature adult, and senior citizen drug use).
- Prevention programs have to be tailored to the characteristics of the audience (e.g., age, gender, ethnicity, extent of drug use).

Levels of Drug Prevention

- **Level 1: Primary Prevention**
  - **Primary drug prevention programs** refer to a very broad range of activities aimed at reducing the risk of drug use among non-users and assuring continued non-use. The emphasis of primary drug prevention programs are aimed at either nonusers who need to be "inoculated" against potential drug use and helping at-risk individuals avoid the development of addictive behaviors. Often targeted to at-risk individuals, neighborhoods, communities, and families.

Levels of Drug Prevention (continued)

- Level 1 Factors:
  - **Intrapersonal factors:** Affective education, values clarification, personal and social skills development (assertiveness and refusal skills), drug information and education
  - **Small group factors:** Peer mentoring, conflict resolution, curriculum infusion, clarification of peer norms, alternatives, strengthening families
  - **Systems level:** Strengthening school-family links, school-community links, and community support systems, media advocacy efforts, reduce alcohol marketing

Levels of Drug Prevention (continued)

- **Level 2: Secondary Prevention**
  - **Secondary drug prevention programs** consist of uncovering potentially harmful substance use prior to the onset of overt symptoms or problems and/or targeting newer drug users with a limited early history of drug use. Overall, the focus is on at-risk groups, such as *early* experimenters having some abuse problems in order to stop the progression to drugs of abuse (similar to "early intervention").

Levels of Drug Prevention (continued)

- Level 2 Programs:
  - Assessment strategies: identification of abuse subgroups and individual diagnoses
  - Early intervention coupled with sanctions
  - Teacher-counselor-parent team approach
  - Developing healthy alternative youth culture
  - Use of recovering role models

Levels of Drug Prevention (continued)

- **Level 3: Tertiary Prevention**
  - **Tertiary drug prevention** programs focus directly on intervention. Tertiary drug prevention targets chemically dependent individuals who need treatment so that further disability is minimized. The primary focus is intervention at an advanced state of drug use/abuse. Very similar to drug abuse treatment.

Notes

Notes

Levels of Drug Prevention (continued)

- Level 3 Programs:
  - Assessment and diagnosis
  - Referral to treatment
  - Case management
  - Reentry into a life without drugs

Levels of Drug Prevention (continued)

- Primary, secondary, and tertiary programs are often used *in combination* because, in most settings, all three types of drug users constitute the targeted population.

Drug Prevention Programs Should be "Pitched" to Specific Audiences

- Non-users
- Early experimenters of drugs
- Non-problem drug users: Those who abuse drugs on occasion, mostly for recreation purposes
- Non-detected, committed, or secret users: Those who abuse drugs and have no interest in stopping
- Problem users
- Former users

Comprehensive Prevention Programs for Drug Use and Abuse

- What are some of the unique characteristics of the following?
  - Harm reduction model
  - Community-based prevention
  - School-based drug prevention
  - School-based prevention through law enforcement
  - Family-based prevention programs

Comprehensive Prevention Programs for Drug Use and Abuse (continued)

- **Harm Reduction:** Practiced in Netherlands and in the United Kingdom. Meets addicts on their own level. Uses an "open door" policy. Addicts are encouraged to take part in prevention and treatment services. Calls for the non-judgmental, non-coercive provision of services and resources to people who use drugs and the communities in which they live to assist them in reducing attendant harm.
- **Community-Based Prevention:** Provide coordinated programs among many agencies and organizations involved in prevention.
- **School-Based Prevention through Law Enforcement:** Grounded in prohibitionist philosophy this approach is devoid of public health perspectives and strategies. Examples include: anti-smoking and zero-tolerance policies, drug searches, and drug testing.

Comprehensive Prevention Programs for Drug Use and Abuse (continued)

- **School-Based Prevention:** Drug education in elementary, junior high, senior high, and college level.
- **Family-Based Prevention:** Stresses the quality of parent-child interaction, communication skill, child management practices, and family management.
- **Individual-Based Drug Prevention and Treatment: Harm Reduction Psychotherapy (HRT):** Based on the belief that alcohol and other drug problems develop in the individual through a unique interaction of biological, psychological, and social factors. It is a non-judgmental therapy approach emphasizing collaboration, respect, and self determination.

Notes

Notes

Drug Education Strategies

- Strategies that focus on and provide drug use/abuse information
- Strategies that stress non-drug-use values, beliefs, and attitudes
- Strategies that emphasize the consequences of drug use (namely, warnings and scare tactics about drug abuse)

Major Drug Prevention Strategies

- **Scare tactic approach:** Drug prevention information based on emphasizing the extreme negative effects of drug use by coercing/warning the audience about the dangers of drug use.
- **Information-only or awareness model:** Assumes that teaching about the harmful effects of drugs will change attitudes about use and abuse.

Major Drug Prevention Strategies (continued)

- **Attitude change model or affective education model:** Assumes people use drugs because of a lack of self-esteem and other personality factors.
- **Social influences model:** Assumes that drug users lack resistance skills. Examples include teaching skills to resist drug use.
- **Ecological or person-in-environment model:** Focuses on the causes of drug use resulting largely from the social environment (drug use and abuse problems among the young are social). This perspective emphasizes that it is important to take into account all of the environments that may have an impact on drug use. Friends, acquaintances, roommates, and classmates in dorms, sororities, and fraternities, at parties, cafes, and nightspots can influence students.

Major Drug Prevention Strategies (continued)

- Major prevention strategies include:
  - Dissemination of drug information
  - Cognitive and behavioral skills training for youth, parents, and professionals, and mass media
  - Mass media programming
  - Grass roots citizen participation
  - Leadership training
  - Policy analysis and reformulation

Making Drug Education Programs More Effective

- Practice deliberate planning
- Review the previous history
- Establish links between the messages conveyed and learned and other aspects of students' life experiences
- Effectively promote programs
- Properly allocate resources
- Constantly evaluate effectiveness of program

Examples of Current Large-Scale Drug Prevention Programs

- **The *BACCHUS* Network:** An organization often found on college and university campuses. Focuses on promoting and disseminating research and effective strategies to help campuses and communities address health and safety issues, primarily alcohol abuse, sexual responsibility, tobacco use, marijuana use, and sexual assault.
- **D.A.R.E. (Drug Abuse Resistance Education):** School-based drug education programs by law enforcement officials.
- **Drug courts:** Courts (e.g., Adult, Veterans, Family Drug, Juvenile, Reentry, and Tribal Courts) designed to focus on *treatment programs* and other options instead of simply incarcerating (jailing) drug offenders. Judges share power with defense counsel, prosecutors, treatment providers, and law enforcement officers at staff meetings in rendering verdicts (decisions) on drug charges.

Notes

Notes

Other Alternatives to Drug Use

- **Alternatives approach:** An approach emphasizing the exploration of positive alternatives to drug abuse, based on replacing the pleasurable feelings experienced from drug use with involvement in social and educational activities. Examples include athletics, exercise, hiking, cultivating hobbies, mountain climbing, and getting involved in other physically or mentally challenging alternatives.

Other Alternatives to Drug Use (continued)

- **Meditation:** A state of consciousness in which there is a constant level of awareness focusing on one object; for example, getting involved in yoga and/or Zen Buddhism.

Natural Mind Approach

- Trading the "high" from drugs for the "high" achieved in meditation. The natural mind approach involves achieving the "high" previously experienced from drugs through meditation *without using any drugs*. Learning to value other "highs" other than experiencing drug "highs."
- *How successful and long-lasting can this approach be?* In response to this question, Andrew Weil (1972, p. 67) stated: "One does not see any long-time meditators give up meditation to become acid heads."

CHAPTER 18

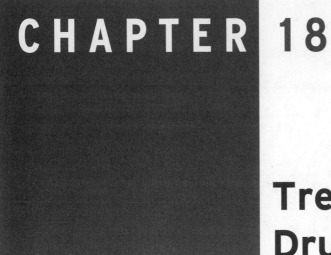

Treating Drug Dependence

The chapter outline provides you with an organizational guide to the topics and ideas presented in this chapter of the text.

Treatment of Addiction
Assessing Addiction Severity and Readiness to Change
Principles of Treatment
Comorbidity
Drug Addiction Treatment in the United States
- Historical Approaches
- General Therapeutic Strategies
- Behavioral Therapies
- Pharmacological Strategies

Key Terms

Define the following terms:

1. **Open meetings** ______________________________
2. **Closed meetings** ______________________________
3. **Therapeutic community** ______________________________
4. **Agonist** ______________________________
5. **Antagonist** ______________________________
6. **Minnesota model** ______________________________
7. **Alcoholics Anonymous** ______________________________
8. **Partial agonist** ______________________________
9. **Co-morbidity** ______________________________

■ Identify

1. Identify five of the 13 NIDA principles that characterize effective addiction treatment.

a. ______________________________

b. ______________________________

c. ______________________________

d. ______________________________

e. ______________________________

2. Identify and discuss three general therapeutic approaches used to treat substance abuse.

a. ______________________________

b. ______________________________

c. ______________________________

3. Identify and discuss three drug abuse treatment strategies that involve specific pharmacological agents.

a. ______________________________

b. ______________________________

c. ______________________________

■ Discussion Questions

1. Discuss the process of assessing addiction severity and readiness to change. ______________________________

____

____

____

2. Describe Alcoholics Anonymous. Why is it difficult to assess its success? ______________________________

____

____

____

3. Describe the Minnesota Model of drug treatment. ______________________________

____

____

____

4. How are pharmacological strategies used to treat drug abuse? Give two examples of these therapies.

____

____

____

5. Discuss the role of co-morbidity in the treatment of drug abuse. ______________________

____

____

____

Notes

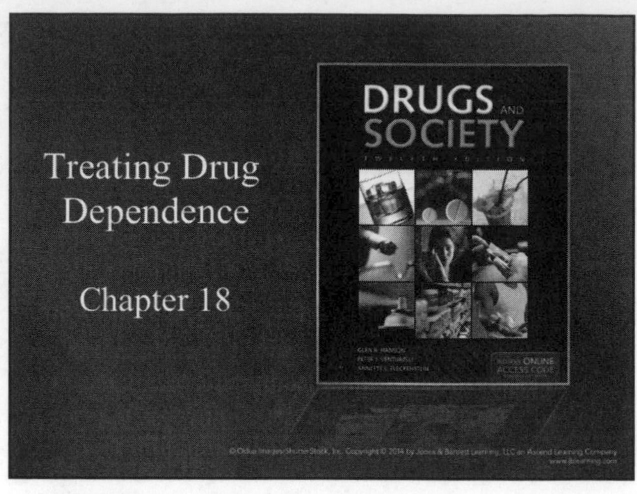

Treatment of Addiction

- Individuals who are addicted to drugs come from all walks of life.
- Many suffer from occupational, social, psychiatric or other medical problems that can make their addictions difficult to treat.
- The severity of addictions varies widely. It is essential to match treatment with the needs of the client.

Treatment of Addiction (continued)

- It is valuable to intervene at the earliest possible stage of addiction with the least restrictive form of appropriate treatment.
- It is important that treatment providers determine the severity of addiction as well as the readiness of an individual to change his or her behavior.

Assessing Addiction Severity and Readiness to Change

- **Addiction Severity Index (ASI):** Among the most widely used assessment instruments in the field.
- The ASI focuses on possible problems in six areas: medical status, employment and support, alcohol and drug use, legal status, family and social relationships, and psychiatric status.
- The ASI provides information that can be used to identify and prioritize which problem areas are most significant and require prompt attention.

Maslow's Hierarchy of Needs

- Includes food, drink, warmth, sleep, and shelter.
- Can be extended to problems including unidentified or inappropriately managed health problems, medication adherence issues, and physical alterations due to drug and/or alcohol dependence.
- Once fundamental needs are addressed, a second level of needs involving security and safety can be addressed including such issues as stability, order, law, and limits.

Prochaska and DiClemente

- Change as a Multistage Process
  - Pre-contemplation
  - Contemplation
  - Preparation
  - Action
  - Maintenance

Notes

Notes

Principles of Treatment

- Variety of approaches to treating addiction
  - Behavioral therapy
  - Counseling
  - Psychotherapy
  - Cognitive therapy
  - Pharmacological therapy
- Successful programs often combine therapies

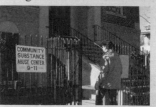

COMMUNITY SUBSTANCE ABUSE CENTER 9-11

Treatment facilities provide a variety of services to people dealing with substance abuse.

Principles of Treatment (continued)

- Many who enter treatment drop out before receiving all of its benefits.
- Successful treatment often requires more than one treatment exposure.
- Relapse rates for addiction resemble those of other chronic diseases, such as diabetes, hypertension, and asthma.

NIDA's Principles of Drug Treatment

- Addiction is a complex but treatable disease that affects brain function and behavior.
- No single treatment is appropriate for all individuals.
- Treatment needs to be readily available.
- Effective treatment attends to multiple needs of the individual, not just to his/her drug use.
- Remaining in treatment for an adequate period is critical.
- Behavioral therapies are the most commonly used forms of drug abuse treatment.

NIDA's Principles of Drug Treatment (continued)

- Medications are an important element of treatment for many patients, especially when combined with counseling and other behavioral therapies.
- An individual's treatment and services plan must be assessed continually and modified as necessary to ensure that it meets his or her changing needs.
- Many drug-addicted individuals also have other mental disorders.
- Medically assisted detoxification is only the first stage of addiction treatment and by itself does little to change long-term drug use.

NIDA's Principles of Drug Treatment (continued)

- Treatment does not need to be voluntary to be effective.
- Drug use during treatment must be monitored continuously, as lapses during treatment do occur.
- Treatment programs should assess patients for the presence of HIV/ AIDS, hepatitis B and C, tuberculosis, and other infectious diseases as well as provide targeted risk-reduction counseling to help patients modify or change behaviors that place them at risk of contracting or spreading infectious diseases.

Other Important Considerations

- The age of the abuser is an important consideration when designing treatment, including both the age of exposure to drugs and the age at which treatment is initiated.
- From birth through early adulthood, the brain undergoes a prolonged process of development during which a behavioral shift occurs such that actions go from being more impulsive to more reflective and reasoned.

Notes

Notes

Other Important Considerations

- The brain areas most closely associated with judgment, decision-making, and self-control undergo a period of rapid development during adolescence.
- Treatment should attend not only to biological distinctions between genders but also to the social and environmental factors that can differentially influence motivations for drug use, treatments that are most effective, reasons for seeking treatment, types of environments where treatment is obtained, and consequences of not receiving treatment.

Other Important Considerations

- Gender-related considerations in the treatment of substance abuse are of importance.
- Criminal justice-involved substance abusers are another population that often benefits from specialized treatment approaches.
- Therapeutic work environments that provide employment for abstinent drug-abusing individuals promote a continued drug-free lifestyle.

Other Important Considerations

- Several factors influence retention in treatment programs, including individual motivation to change drug-using behavior and degree of support from family and friends.
- Pressure from employers, the criminal justice system, and/or extensions of the court (i.e., child protective services) can be important.

Notes

Comorbidity

- A condition where two or more illnesses occur in the same person, simultaneously or sequentially.
- *Comorbidity* also suggests interactions between the illnesses that affect the course and prognosis of both.

Comorbidity (continued)

- Comorbidity between drug addiction and other mental illnesses is common.
- Mental illnesses can sometimes lead to substance abuse and addiction in that individuals sometimes abuse drugs to self-medicate an underlying medical condition.

Comorbidity (continued)

- The high incidence of co-morbidity between substance abuse disorders and other mental illnesses does not mean that one necessarily caused the other.
- Effective treatment of individuals with co-morbid substance abuse and mental illnesses requires accurate diagnosis of both conditions.

Notes

Comorbidity (continued)

- Several fundamental barriers impede treatment of co-morbid disorders.
- Often, one professional background is broad enough to address the full range of problems presented by patients.
- A bias exists in some substance abuse treatment facilities against using any pharmacological intervention, including those necessary to treat serious mental illnesses, such as depression.

Drug Addiction Treatment in the United States

- According to SAMSHA, in 2011, 21.6 million persons needed treatment for an illicit drug or alcohol use problem.
- However, in 2011, only 2.3 million persons received treatment at a specialty facility

Reported Reasons Treatment Not Obtained

- Lack of health coverage and could not afford cost.
- A lack of readiness to stop using
- A possible negative effect on job
- Persons had health coverage but did not cover treatment or did not cover cost
- A lack of transportation or inconvenience
- Persons did not know where to go for treatment
- Perception that it might cause neighbors/community to have negative opinion
- A lack of time for treatment

Important Consideration

- Research has demonstrated that treatment is far less expensive than simply incarcerating addicts.

Mental Health Parity and Addiction Equity Act

- Requires group health insurance plans (involving greater than 50 insured employees) that offer coverage for mental illness and substance use disorders to provide those benefits in a no more restrictive manner than all other medical/surgical procedures covered by the plan.

Historic Approaches to Treatment

- Alcoholics Anonymous
  - Open vs. Closed Meetings
  - Al-Anon, Alateen
- Minnesota Model

Notes

Notes

General Therapeutic Strategies

- Some are individualized and some are group-based.
- Not all treatment programs fit perfectly into any one category
- Include short-term inpatient, long-term inpatient and outpatient therapy

Medical Detoxification

- The process of safely managing the acute physical symptoms of withdrawal associated with stopping drug use
- Medications including benzodiazepines and other sedatives are often utilized
- Can be medically necessary because untreated withdrawal from some agents can be fatal.
- Although sometimes referred to as a distinct treatment modality, it is more appropriately considered a precursor to treatment

Therapeutic Communities (TCs)

- The best-known residential treatment model
- Focus on the "resocialization" of the individual and use the program's entire community (e.g., staff, other residents) as important treatment components
- Planned lengths of stay in TCs are often between 6 and 12 months.
- TCs often offer comprehensive services, which can include employment training on site.

Behavioral Therapies

- Cognitive Behavioral Therapy
- Contingency Management (CM) Interventions/ Motivational Incentives
- Community Reinforcement Approach (CRA) Plus Vouchers
- Motivational Enhancement Therapy (MET)
- The Matrix Model
- 12-Step Facilitation

Pharmacological Therapies

- Methadone
- Naloxone and Naltrexone
- Nicotine Replacement
- Clonidine
- Antabuse
- Acomprosate and Topiramate

Methadone

- An opioid agonist
- Long-acting synthetic opiate medication administered orally for a sustained period at a dosage sufficient to prevent opiate withdrawal and decrease craving
- Patients stabilized on adequate, sustained dosages of methadone can function normally.

Notes

Notes

Naloxone

- A short-acting opioid antagonist, naloxone (Narcan), is often used in the emergency treatment of opioid overdoses.

Naltrexone

- A long-acting synthetic opioid antagonist
- Individuals must be opioid-free for several days before taking naltrexone in order to avoid withdrawal symptoms.
- An extended release preparation of the drug (Vivitrol) have been shown to reduce relapse to problem drinking in some patients.

Nicotine Replacement

- Nicotine gum, transdermal patches, nasal sprays and inhalers

Notes

Clonidine

- Clonidine is not addictive and does not cause euphoria, but it does block cravings for some drugs.

Antabuse

- Used for treating alcoholics.
- Causes nausea, vomiting, flushing, and anxiety if an individual consumes alcohol while taking the drug.
- A deterrent drug.

Acomprosate and Topiramate

- Novel mechanism of action
- Act on the glutamate and gamma-aminobutyric acid (GABA) neurotransmitter systems.

Notes

Drug Addiction Treatment Act

- Subutex and Suboxone tablets approved for the treatment of opiate dependence by specially trained physicians. Accordingly, the drugs can be prescribed in an office setting and, therefore, can provide greater access to patients needing treatment.

Buprenorphine

- A partial agonist at opioid receptors.
- Reduces or eliminates withdrawal symptoms associated with opioid dependence but generally does not produce the euphoria and sedation caused by other opioids.
- Available in two formulations—Subutex, which contains only buprenorphine, and Suboxone, which contains both buprenorphine and naloxone.